Footprin
The Sand

To Liz.

God Bless

Crawford.

Crawford Buchan

chipmunkapublishing
the mental health publisher

Published by
Chipmunkapublishing
United Kingdom

http://www.chipmunkapublishing.com

ISBN   978-1-84991-992-0

Chipmunkapublishing gratefully acknowledge the support of Arts Council England.

From Bipolar Heaven to Hell and Back

This is the amazing story of one mans continued quest to prove that God exists despite his bipolar disorder. Crawford Buchan is dedicating his life to proving that God exists and as you will discover when you read the book he is not about to pass up on the wonderful gift he has been given as he is willing to make the ultimate sacrifice if called upon to prove that God does in fact exist.

The front cover is designed by Isabel Christie a friend from Letham St Marks Church.

The names of most of the characters that have shaped my life have been changed to protect their identity.

The book is dedicated to all those people who know what it is like to go to sleep and wake in a darkness that no light can penetrate. Remember this if nothing else.

'This is the day the LORD has made; Let us rejoice and be glad in it'

PREFACE

The main requirement when reading this book is an open mind. I have never and will never try and force my beliefs on to someone else. Like everything in life we have to make our own choices. It is similar to my addiction to cigarettes which I have for the time being managed to kick even if this was as a result of complications during brain surgery and not down to a personal choice. I would however probably recommend nicotine patches before going down the brain surgery route! The names of most of the people in this book have been changed to protect their identities.

Just in case you are in any doubt about what I'm trying to say in this book then I will make it very clear. I think that God who created this wonderful world and all the creatures that live in it has come to the point where he has said enough is enough. No longer does he want to see thousands killed in numerous wars and civil unrest, children dying from starvation when we throw away tonnes of food on a daily basis. Murder, rape, child abuse and terrorist attacks are now so common we have become desensitised to it on the evening news. How does he change this catalogue of destruction? The only way is to make people aware that their actions will carry consequences as God does not like sin. He gave his only Son so that he could be sacrificed for our sins yet still we have not learned. Up until very recently I believed the only way to do this was for me to prove that God exists and with this prove to people that there was a heaven and indeed a hell. I say recently because now although I know there is a heaven I'm not convinced that hell exists. You may then ask what the consequences of our own sinful actions are when judgement day comes. Well I believe that these actions will mean we are not given the keys to heaven and eternal life and that death will just be the end of everything we know and feel. That in its self should act as a sufficient deterrent.

Now you may ask as I do every day why have I been chosen to deliver this message to the world. What makes me so special and the answer to that is simple. Nothing. Like everybody else I'm a sinner who prays for forgiveness every day. I'm not a minister so I can't explain the Bible to you or quote relevant passages. I'm just a normal guy from a small city in Scotland whose whole life's journey has been in preparation to deliver this message to those of us who have chosen to forget it. Now just as it was our choice to forget it we can also choose to refresh our memories as a new year begins and I guarantee that good times will come if you do. Do not expect too much though as I'm just a normal guy who goes to watch the Saints (St. Johnstone) on a Saturday and yes I do sometimes swear at the subpar performances! I can't perform miracles either so don't expect us to win the SPL any time soon!

GOD BLESS

CHAPTER ONE

My name is Crawford Buchan and I'm forty three years old. I was diagnosed with Dystonia and in particular Spasmodic Torticollis in 1997. I was diagnosed with bipolar disorder a year later. I was born in Perth Royal Infirmary on December 20th 1969. In fact the maternity ward is now only five hundred yards from where I'm typing this book and I often think that if they had dropped me of the delivery table I could have crawled here in a couple of years! I am the youngest of three children with a brother Scott in Glasgow, who is a year older than me and a sister, Shuna in London, who is a year older than him. I have thought a lot recently about the old joke which suggested I may not have been a mistake but just an accident and I have probably thought the former is nearer the truth but maybe I will explain my reasoning behind that later.

My first home was in the village of Pitcairngreen which was a typical small village with all the houses circling the green which was used for the usual village fetes and local football matches. Our house as far as I can remember was like most dotted round the green but I do remember the distinctive smell of the chicken farm that it backed on to. My early childhood was fairly uneventful and I remember it to be a happy one.

The only major drama in those early years happened the day before I was due to start primary school. I was on my tricycle going down a small hill beside the local guest house a couple of hundred yards from my front door. In my right hand I was carrying a runner bean cane (a bamboo cane used to tie runner bean stems to) and as I pedalled down the hill I was totally unaware of the imminent danger the boulders at the bottom of the slope posed. My front wheel careered into the middle boulder and my right hand came of the handle bars towards my open mouth. The bamboo cane entered my mouth hit the back wall, snapped and the top half penetrated up through the top pallet of my mouth, the bottom half came back down into my throat. I certainly can't remember any pain as I was probably in a state of shock but the coalman carried me back to my house where I was met at the front door by my mum who looked at me in horror. The two pieces of cane protruding from my bloody mouth did not paint a pretty picture. I can't remember much about what happened next but I was rushed to the local hospital where the pieces of cane were removed and my upper pallet stitched up and I was allowed home a couple of days later. However when I got home I was eating some soup when I dropped my spoon and started to slur my speech which alarmed my mother. The slurred speech was nothing out of the ordinary but I definitely didn't like to waste food. I was rushed to Ninewell's Hospital in Dundee where they removed a blood clot on my brain. This was removed with the minimum of fuss although I did manage to miss the first two weeks of primary school and have been trying to catch up ever since!

The village primary was unsurprisingly called Pitcairngreen Primary although technically it should really have been called Almondbank Primary as it was nearer to Almondbank. It was a small school sitting in the middle of the large slope which led up from Almondbank and over the top to Pitcairngreen. It probably only had about 120 pupils at most and they were divided between seven classes. There was a playground at one end with a shed at the top to shelter from the cold winds in winter and a netball court at the other which backed on to the playing field which couldn't really be used for any games as it sloped so much from left to right. Mind you that didn't stop the school sports day being held there every year. My years there were happy ones with lots of funny stories but also for the first time in my life I felt the pressure to succeed and this would dog me for another thirty years.

Despite the many good times at primary school the Buchan family had created many myths over the years and these at times did result in us being placed quite high up the pecking order when the bullies were bored of the usual suspects and needed another relatively easy target. The myths were in a way understandable at that age. We had a very large garden and my father had hired a private golf coach for me so this meant we actually had our own nine hole golf course. Our neighbour's daughter was going out with a commercial helicopter pilot and he used to land in the field at the bottom of our garden which meant we also owned a helicopter.

These myths were I think further enforced when first my sister and then my brother in consecutive years were awarded the schools highest honour at the school prize giving. The award for academic achievement above all others was known as the Dux of the school and now I was the only Buchan standing in the way of a glorious hat-trick. All major school functions, music classes, assemblies were held in the school gymnasium. At the prize giving the expectant parents would sit on chairs at the back and the pupils would sit crossed legged at the front. The Dux was always the last prize to be awarded and I waited with hope and quite a lot of dread for the results to be announced. 'And the Dux of the school is' I didn't really here my name being read out but I can remember feeling as if it was an awful long way from where I was sitting to the front of the small gymnasium and it seemed to take for ever to get there. I wasn't even half way there when the first cries of 'fix' started to ring out followed by 'three little Dux' 'Quack, quack ,quack' and they were not only from the usual pupils as parents were now joining in. I accepted the award and scuttled back to my place as quickly as I could. Why had I put so much pressure on myself to win something that in the end brought me no joy whatsoever? When I met my parents and the two other Dux's after my father suggested we go to the local pub for a meal to celebrate my achievement but I thought he must have booked the table beforehand for some reason and despite his good intentions this only served to reinforce my belief that the award actually was a fix. Throughout my life I would put virtually all of my achievements down to external forces such as bribes and back handers from my Dad and therefore I never really got any joy from them and I certainly didn't take any of the credit for them.

I started secondary school in late August 1991 at Perth Grammar School. The word Grammar seemed to give the school some air of superiority but it probably had the worst reputation of any of the local secondary schools. It was situated in an area of Perth between Muirton and North Muirton. Now where the line between the two areas started and finished was unclear to me but to the people who lived there it seemed to be of greater importance. The school was home to some fourteen hundred pupils which was a big step up from the one hundred or so that had attended Pitcairngreen Primary but I managed to settle in without too many problems. I made friends easily and although I didn't have that many I could rely on those I had. Most of my friends were more academically inclined which suited me as in the long run it meant that we were not surrounded by trouble as some were. I certainly wasn't near the top of the food chain or for that fact the 'in' crowd but I got by and getting by in Perth Grammar was a safe place to be. The weak proved easy prey and for four years you could see the vultures picking at their lifeless corpses. I was happy to remain largely anonymous and get on with my school work. If you wanted to learn then the Grammar was a good school with a lot of competent teachers who were willing to help you get to where you wanted to be. My best subject was and had always been mathematics. Unlike life I liked the idea of turning the handle and getting an answer that was either right or wrong. There was no room for grey in maths, only black or white and I think I craved the clarity and logic of the subject. Also the best teacher in the school, or at least I thought, was my math's teacher. A large red cheeked, always cheery man Mr Davidson seemed to be consumed by his passion for maths and he wanted to make sure that all his pupils fulfilled their potential in the subject. Figures came extremely easy to me and this made the subjects appeal even greater as I loved things that I was good at and could show off my skills in. I got ninety eight percent in the maths higher prelim exam, only missing out on the perfect score because I misread a multiple choice question. However pride often comes before a fall and I only got a B in the actual exam which was very embarrassing after being awarded the maths prize earlier in the year. I felt really bad for Mr Davidson who gallantly tried to fight my corner by appealing the mark based on my prelim score but unfortunately this was in vain. I would however go some way to repaying all his patience when I went to St Andrews University to study mathematics and statistics.

I'm not sure why I chose St. Andrews to continue my educational journey. It was probably because it was a relatively small town compared to the big city options of Glasgow and Edinburgh. It would not appear to be such a leap into the unknown and also my big sister was already there and she only had glowing reports from her time there. Last but by no means least were the eight golf courses I would have access to at the ridiculously low rate of £42 per year and yes that did include unlimited play on the old course! Oh and by the way they also offered my preferred academic course, Mathematics and Statistics! For the first two years I was in halls of residence and by pure luck I was allocated Hamilton Halls which is the big red building behind the eighteenth green of the Old Course Golf Course. The holy grail for golfers, of any ability. I could finish my dinner and walk on to the first tee of the most famous golf course in the world without a sideways glance from anybody looking out from the St Andrews club house. I managed to get myself a place on the golf team so we got to play some courses away from home as well but I lost more games than I won as far as I can remember. In my third year I moved out into a flat with 3 other friends which was an eye opener as I now had to cook, clean and do all those other things you take for granted when you live in halls like not having to pay any bills.

I returned to the easy life in my final year as I wanted to concentrate on studying for my finals so I returned to Hamilton Halls. As a final year student and with the rooms being allocated in alphabetic order I got first choice of any room in the entire Hall. I chose a third floor room with a balcony looking over the eighteenth green.

Despite having first choice of my room it was in fresher's week that the blackness in my life really began. I had been drinking heavily as most students tended to do in fresher's week as you are reacquainted with pals after the summer holidays and you make new pals with the students that are just starting out on their own academic journey. Maybe they should rename it refreshers week as large quantities of all sorts of beverages are drunk by the old and newcomers. I was no different but I awoke one morning to find that I had a slight tremor in both hands but more noticeably in my left hand. No wonder I hear you say and I did at first think that this was some form of the DT's kicking in but it didn't go away even when I had stopped drinking completely. We always had fish and chips with peas on a Friday in the halls and it was always my favourite but one Friday I couldn't even eat the peas as my fork was shaking so much that they were disappearing off in all directions.

After waiting for several alcohol free weeks hoping the tremors would pass I realised this was not going to happen and in fact if anything they had got worse so I decided to make an appointment with a local GP. He diagnosed anxiety and stress and prescribed a course of beta blockers to calm my shakes. Now I am not denying the fact that stress exists in everyday life and manifests itself in many ways but I up to that point in my life had been stress free and it was very difficult for me to accept that something in my mind was causing these tremors. Never the less I took the medication and for a time the psychological effect of having them as a safety net seemed to work but for the most part nothing changed and I just battled on. However this imperfection was causing my mood to sink lower and lower and I would only really find out how low two years later when I attempted suicide for the first time.

The day after my graduation two university friends and I headed off around the world. This was certainly not an all-expenses paid trip. I left with only 52 US dollars in my pocket for the year so I knew when I left that I needed a job as soon as possible. We went to Boston first as this is where my sister was staying with her American fiancée who she had met at St. Andrews. Paul the piper and Stuart the drummer did not have to get a job as quickly as me because due to their musical talents they were making money busking on Boston Common. The first job I got was collecting door to door for the 'Massachusetts Campaign to Clean Up Hazardous Waste' which was a charity based in Boston and believe me it wasn't easy to get people to part with the minimum amount required each night to ensure that I did not lose my job. We were staying in a flat that had been paid for up to the end of the month by its previous tenant but had already had the power supply turned off. I slept on the bear wooden floor and we used candles when it got dark until completely out of the blue this man turned up and put the power back on for which we rewarded him with a six pack of beer! The main event for me in that flat was I lost my virginity too a very nice twenty nine year old woman whose name has escaped me for the moment. I know this was fairly late in life but I have to say my first time was nothing spectacular and I don't know why I had been so desperate to lose my virginity come to think of it. It was not the ladies fault as she could tell I was inexperienced even though I did lie and say it was my second time! Believe me I can guarantee that it was not memorable for her although it may well have been the worst sex she had ever had for all I know!

I will not bore you with all my stories about our travels across America, Hawaii, Australia and New Zealand. I will save them for another book! The good thing was that during my travels the tremor in my hand disappeared. I put this down to the fact that for the first time in my life I was in total control and I was responsible for my own passport and where I was going to sleep each night and how I was going to pay for that and my next meal and next beer. Needless to say I had an amazing time travelling but it was with some dread that I thought about coming back to the UK and in the end this would be justified.

Almost as the plane touched back down in Scotland my tremors returned and they were not just restricted to my hands. They had moved to the side of my neck causing it to pull to the right in painful spasms that I could not control. None of my family could actually see the tremors but this didn't matter to me as I could feel them and I thought this meant everybody else could see them. I tried to tell my mother that I could not live with this imperfection but she did not realise that I was meaning this literally.

One evening when my parents had gone to bed I poured myself a pint of water and proceeded to take 50 or so extra strength Hedex pills before going to bed. Now some people would say this was just a cry for help but they would be wrong. A cry for help only becomes a suicide attempt when it succeeds. The other cliché that always comes out of people's mouths is that suicide is the' cowards way out'. Let me tell you that when you do something that could end your own life it is not because you are a coward. It is because you feel so low that you just can't carry on anymore even if you are quite aware that the act itself will devastate your loved ones permanently. Try and put yourself in the suicidal person's shoes for once. You know how much they love their family and children yet they still feel this is their only option so that may give you some idea of how bad they feel.

I was lying in my bed and I thought my heart may come out of my chest it was beating so fast. So much for just dropping off to sleep and never waking up again. I ran to the toilet and threw up and because I had thrown up I started to realise that this attempt was not going to work. I jumped in my mother's jeep and started to drive to the hospital checking in my mirror that no lights had come on in the house as the car wheels spun on the gravel drive. I drove down to Perth Royal Infirmary as quickly as I could, stopping once on the way down to throw up again. I parked the car and walked into the accident and emergency department. I stopped the first nurse that I saw and explained to her what I had done but I don't think she really believed me until I threw up again. It was not long before I was admitted. The first treatment was a charcoal drip which is not very pleasant as you end up throwing up black vomit for several hours. Fortunately it was the nursing staff who phoned my parents to let them know what I had done as I don't think I could really face telling them. They were really shocked of course although it did surprise me just how much as I thought that they might have had some idea about how low I was feeling even if no one in our family ever discussed their feelings. I think I was offered the chance to speak to a psychiatrist about what I had attempted to do and I may even have seen one at Murray Royal Hospital but he only prescribed mild anti-depressants which were really no good as they were not going to help with my tremors which were at the root of my low mood.

This suicide attempt like most things in my family was just swept under the carpet as if it never happened apart from having to promise my Dad that I would never try it again. That was a promise I should never have made. Two months later I started my accountancy training with Ernst & Young in Glasgow. The one thing I said I would never be at University was an accountant as I had it in my head that it would be extremely boring. As I hadn't done accountancy at university I had to do all the Professional exams which weren't too taxing if you excuse the pun. The other two exams TPC1 and TPC2 were much more of a test and even the carrot of a one thousand pound bonus for a first time pass each time did not mean they would be plain sailing. However despite fears to the contrary I passed first time and qualified as an accountant towards the end of 1995. Now I can't say that I enjoyed my time at Ernst & Young as my tremors continued to get more visible and my neck was now pulling further and further over to the right. These spasms were always worse during stressful jobs at work.

I think that is why I decided to resign immediately after I received my accountancy qualification and go travelling again with two friends from work, Peter and Paul. This time we headed of for Whistler in Canada for the ski season. We were able to afford some better accommodation than the last time I went travelling as we had all saved some money for our trip. We stayed first at the Boot Bar which was really like a youth hostel. Unfortunately the girl that I had been seeing in Glasgow before I left had three children one of whom had chicken pox. To my horror I found out from my Mum that I had never had this and it was only when I was in my bunk bed during our first week away that my first spot burst. We spent three months in Whistler although Peter went home after a few weeks as travelling wasn't for him. It was just a pity he didn't think to tell us he wasn't coming back after he had flown home for a family funeral! After Whistler we flew to Los Angeles and then went island hoping in Hawaii before making another trip to New Zealand. We took the Kiwi Experience bus tour as I had taken this in 1991 and had a great time. I had a great time again and it was on the bus that I met Mary who I would have an up and down relationship with for several months and this even continued when I came back to the UK. Mary was a stunning girl who was really way out of my league looks wise but she was not nearly as nice on the inside at times especially to me. But like a mug I kept going back for more punishment.

After a couple of months in New Zealand we went over to Australia where Paul and I both got jobs working for Citibank as debt collectors. We would phone people up about their overdue credit card, mortgage and car payments. I did this for the whole year before leaving to spend a few weeks doing the OZ experience bus tour up the East coast of Australia. This was the Australian equivalent of the Kiwi Experience and I had a great time again. After coming back to Sydney I arranged to spend a couple of weeks in Bali on the way back to Scotland. Just like before my old symptoms started to return almost as the wheels of the plane touched down at Heathrow.

I arrived back in March 1997 and despite my returning tremors I had used up most of my funds travelling so it was time to get a job. I managed to get one very quickly as an accountant for a company based just outside Edinburgh. I have to say the first few days working there were very stressful and as a result my neck was absolute agony pulling to the right hand side. As the symptoms were still put down to stress by a doctor who was now prescribing without even seeing me in person, I was now taking 7 valium at one time, working a fourteen hour day and driving between Edinburgh and Perth every day.

I was still in contact with Mary and she basically invited herself up one weekend to celebrate her birthday giving my work colleagues the impression she was my fiancée for some reason. Anyway she ended up snogging one of my work colleagues which was very embarrassing for me and it did little to help with my low mood. In fact when she got back to the house where we were staying I explained that I couldn't take the pain in my neck anymore and had been considering killing myself by crashing my car on the way back from work one day. I think she thought I was just sounding off because she had got off with one of my work mates but to tell you the truth that was an irrelevance compared to the pain in my neck which I couldn't cope with any longer.

I went to work on the Monday and we had a team building day organised at the Marriott Hotel near where we worked. It was the day after Princess Di had died so I remember it for that reason too. By the time I left work I had basically decided that I was going to go through with my plan to crash my car but I didn't know if I would have the guts to do it or the opportunity as I had to make sure there were no other cars close to me when I did what I was going to do. I remember driving out of the hotel car park and for some reason I thought that one of my colleagues was going to run out in front of me and shout "Don't do it" but off course they didn't and so I continued the drive home. I was now at the top of the steep hill that is on the dual carriage way 3 miles before Perth and my heart was starting to beat very fast. There is a bad corner at the bottom of this hill where the camber throws your car off if you are going too fast. I calmly released my seatbelt as I thought that any chance of survival would be taken away if I did not have my belt on. I put my foot on the accelerator as I approached the corner and when I had reached 90 miles an hour I checked that there were no cars behind me in my rear view mirror.

It was all clear so I grabbed the steering wheel and with all my strength pulled it to the left. The forward momentum of the car did not like this sudden change in direction and it took a lot of strength to keep the wheel turning left but eventually the car gave in and it started to roll on to its side. There was no going back now. I think I must have been knocked out as the car began to roll because my next memory was of me lying face down in some gravel at the side of the road. A following car must have stopped as I also remember hearing the driver say 'oh shit' as he came over the crash barrier to where the wrecked car and I were now lying. He must have phoned the various emergency services as the next thing I can remember is going to hospital in the speeding ambulance and being wheeled into the recovery room or maybe it was the assessment room as they did seem to be assessing my injuries. I was still complaining about the pain in my neck but I soon realised that I must have badly damaged my ankle as one of the nurses said 'how can he complain about his neck when his ankle is in that state'. My injuries were not life threatening amazingly but I had a compound dislocated fracture of the ankle that had been so severe that the fire service had straightened it at the scene to prevent me losing my foot. I didn't know it at the time but I also had an even more severe injury to my shoulder. I found out later that when the car flipped it had hit a farm off road propelling it into the air to a height of approximately seventy feet and I had been thrown out of the front windscreen landing on my shoulder on the gravel completely obliterating my right shoulder ball. The only thing that saved me was that I didn't have my seatbelt on as the top of the car was down to the accelerator pedals. I also now know now that someone was watching over me and keeping me safe.

The surgeons did a marvellous job putting me back together and they even managed to rebuild my shoulder ball with some mesh and a couple of screws. I was in hospital for about three weeks but during all this time I was still complaining of the pain in my neck and eventually as nothing had come up in the x-rays I was referred to a neurologist. She looked at me for approximately fifteen seconds and said that I had Dystonia. Even though I had no idea what Dystonia was I responded by saying 'Yes' and clenching my fist in triumph. Finally I had been told that these tremors and spasms were not down to stress but were due to a physical condition called Dystonia which was a fairly rare neurological condition that causes abnormal movements and postures because of uncontrollable spasms. The form that I had was Spasmodic Torticollis which causes the neck to pull to one side. Now after fifteen years of pain caused by Dystonia I don't know if I would still have said 'yes' if I'd known a bit more about the condition and the pain and discomfort it can cause.

The neurologist wasted no time on starting me on the most commonly used treatment for Spasmodic Torticollis which was and still is injections of Botox or Botulinum Toxin into the muscles in the neck. These injections were not very pleasant but over the years I would get so used to them that they were no longer painful. The aim of the injections is to try and paralyse the muscles in the neck which are in spasm but I have found over the years that the success of these was very hit or miss. I was also given a course of nerve painkillers to take but they again had little or no affect. My Dad realised that the crash was probably not an accident and asked me if this was the case. My response of "fuck it" confirmed what he had been thinking but the police who investigated it just put it down as an accident and when they came into hospital to inform me of that you could see that they were amazed I had got out with as little damage as I had. The nurses also thought it was down to a car accident until Mary phoned them up to tell them that she thought it was suicide as I had told her about the exact circumstances of the crash before they happened. I don't know if she did this so I could get some psychiatric treatment or because she felt I had done it because she had snogged one of my work colleagues on a works night out. Mary was a stunner but believe me she was not nearly nice enough for me to kill myself over.

I left hospital in September and there began my long road to recovery. I was in a wheelchair for about three months and because of the delicate surgery needed to rebuild my shoulder I was not allowed to move my right arm any more than a few inches at a time. I spent a lot of time on the exercise bike and in the hydro therapy pool building up my strength. By the time I was allowed to move my arm again the muscles had weakened so much that I could not lift a 1 kilo weight. During all this rehabilitation my neck was even more painful and not responding to any of the treatments which was slowly grinding me down day by day.

My mood had been low for weeks even if I probably hadn't admitted as much to myself. One evening as I walked back to my bedroom in my parent's house I noticed that the light was on in my old bedroom. I had been using the back bedroom since my attempted suicide nine months earlier. My actual bedroom was the middle one downstairs and this still contained everything I had collected since I was a child. I don't know if the light had been left on by my parents but I certainly couldn't remember being in that room for weeks. The light and the open door seemed to be pulling me towards it with some invisible magnetic force. It was as if I didn't have any choice but to enter the room and to be perfectly honest although a little scared by this phenomenon I was also curious to find out what it wanted. I entered cautiously through the door somehow relieved that there was nobody there as I was half expecting to see some shrouded figure. My senses were now standing on edge and my eyes scanned the room like an eagle looking for its next prey. I scanned all my various books on the bookshelf's and they were all mostly about sport and I thought that it would be a selfish act to take one of these to read. I had almost given up hope of finding something meaningful when my eyes were caught by a tiny white book in the middle of the bookshelf. It was not a book I could ever remember being there and that made it stand out even more. I picked it up and as the pages fell open in my hand I realised that it was a very small white New Testament Bible. This was even more surprising to me as apart from Sunday School which Mum used to take at Tibbermore Church I had not been the religiously inclined and my brother and I had eventually been barred from Sunday School for fighting! The bible had fallen open at Matthew Chapter 25 Paragraphs 14-30 'The Parable of the Talents' and I started to read this absorbing every word as if it would be the last I would read. Now I am not a minister so my translation of the Bible may and probably is flawed but this is how I deciphered this Parable.

God gives all of us gifts/talents and he gives some of us more gifts than others. In the parable he gives his faithful servant five gifts and he goes away and uses these gifts to the best of his abilities. When he returns God is happy with his faithful servant and rewards him with another five gifts and allows him to live his life in the joy of the Lord.

God gives another faithful servant two gifts and the servant goes away and uses these two gifts to the best of his abilities. When he returns God is pleased with his faithful servant and rewards him with another two gifts and allows him to live his life in the joy of the Lord.

God gives his last servant one gift but the servant buries this gift in the ground in case he loses it. When he returns and tells God what he has done God is angry with him and takes the gift from him and gives it to the servant who had five talents as he used them most wisely and this servant will be banished to the place where there is great gnashing of teeth which I thought must be hell.

After reading this passage my excitement was so great and the feelings so intense I had to stop myself from running upstairs and waking my parents to tell them of the miracle that had just taken place in their home. Instead I contained myself by writing on a piece of paper:-

Mum, you are right. You believe. I believe. We believe.

Maybe I should call Mr Bain first! Mr Bain was our minister.

I left the Bible on the piece of paper on the kitchen table so that my Mum would see it when she came downstairs in the morning and returned to bed in a state of excitement feeling that for once the world was a great place to be and that I couldn't wait for tomorrow to begin. Usually I loved sleeping as it was the only place where I could dream far away from reality and without the pain of my Dystonia but that night I only wanted morning to come so that I could share my news with the world.

I woke early and had already had two coffees before my mother came downstairs in her dressing gown. I showed her the bible and explained to her what had happened the night before. Although she seemed happy for me she advised me not to tell my father as he may not understand the magnitude of my proclamation. She also didn't seem to understand that God had found me and I think that she thought that her troubled son had found God in his time of need. Despite the rather lacklustre reaction to my news I was still full of the joys of life and for some reason I thought I better document everything that happened during the day in case someday I was asked to prove that God existed. I started to write down the times and dates of small irrelevant things that happened. I would be watching golf on TV and write down 3.45pm, Colin Montgomerie bunkered at the fourteenth or during the football 4.35pm throw in to Manchester United near the corner flag. Everything had to be logged and recorded and I carried on in this manner for the next two days although I can't say that my parents noticed any real difference in my behaviour or if they did they certainly didn't say so.

By the second night the lack of sleep and the constant thoughts racing through my mind were starting to not only confuse me but also make me question the reality of what had happened previously. I knew something was not quite right and despite the fear of asking for help I felt that I had to do something. I made my way up the stairs to my parent's room trying to make as little noise as possible as it was now in the early hours of the morning. I knocked gingerly on the door and like a frightened school boy opened it. I had never really asked for help like this before so I didn't know what sort of reaction I would get. It seemed like something far bigger than saying I had toothache or a really sore throat. My mother was sitting up in bed looking at me intently and rather worriedly at the far end of the room. My Dad was standing at the side of the bed and he looked sternly at me. "I think I need help". My words seemed to take an eternity to travel to the other end of the room and even then the delayed reaction added to my feelings of fear.

The words seemed to land like a current of electricity on my Dads ears as suddenly he came towards me until his face was only inches from mine and he said:-

'You fucking selfish bastard'.

CHAPTER TWO

I was now very scared and those feelings I used to get when I was a little boy and had done something wrong came flooding back. I rushed back down the stairs and went back to the refuge of my room. I lay on the bed trying to make sense of what had just happened. My breathing was very quick and shallow and was getting noticeably worse to the point where I was starting to find it very difficult to catch my breath. I tried to call out for my Mum and Dad but I was unable to shout out because I couldn't draw a breath. I was now even more afraid as I started to hyper- ventilate and I could not get my breathing to slow down.

It was at this moment that I really thought that I was going to die. As I lay on the bed I looked to the left to where the window was and I could only see a blinding light. Now this could well have been car headlights coming up the drive but it wasn't accompanied by the sound of wheels on gravel. I turned to the window on the right of the bedroom and again there was a blinding light but this was more terrifying as there was no road on this side of the house and therefore no logical explanation for the light unless this was how I was going to die and this was God's light. I hadn't envisaged that I would die this way, gasping for breath lying on my bed but maybe I had pushed my luck once too often and this was my time. No sooner had the lights appeared than they vanished which was even more frightening as I now felt totally alone and my breathing was not improving. However as the lights faded I felt that there was less chance of me dying on this particular night. It is difficult to explain what the rest of that night was like but for the entire night, probably some eight or so hours I could not catch my breath yet despite this it was the most exhilarating night of my entire life.

When my fear of dying had subsided I had this overwhelming feeling that I was not alone anymore and I had been embraced by God. For the rest of the night I was shown how painful and difficult my life was going to be. I was not shown the exact details of every day but just snippets of what might happen which included the fact that I may be paralysed from the waist down as I could not move my legs and hence that is why even though I was continually gasping for air I could not go and get help. At times this view in to what the future may hold was terrifying and very daunting as this was not going to be an easy ride but after I had been shown all the pain and suffering I was given a glimpse of how wonderful my life could be after this if I was willing to accept all the tests that I would have to endure before entering the promised land.

When my Mum and Dad eventually came in to check on me the next morning I was still having trouble breathing but I made sure Mum looked into my eyes so that she could recognise that her son was very much still here. They must have phoned the doctor because it was not long before the local GP was looking over me. I think Mum must have also called Reverend Jim Simpson because he was also in my room and he being a man of the church did a much better job of getting my breathing back to normal than the doctor did. Another Doctor who I had never met before also came out to the house and I now know he was a psychiatrist from the local psychiatric hospital in Perth called Murray Royal Hospital. I told Rev Simpson and the psychiatrist what happened the previous night and at no point did it ever cross my mind that they didn't actually believe me. I had been a believer in God for only three days so this was all very new to me and because I now knew how powerful God was I had just assumed that everybody else was in on his grand scheme. I spent the morning talking to the GP and I even hit a few golf balls into the neighbouring farmer's field. I'm not sure but I think a plane flew overhead and the GP told me how he had started having flying lessons out at Scone aerodrome. Even when Mum was asking me what clothes I wanted to take with me I still didn't realise what was happening. I said it didn't matter because the fact that I could now prove that God existed was far more important than what I was going to wear. I think I got in the car with the GP and the psychiatrist but it may have been my Mum who drove us. I just thought that they had believed me and that they were taking me to a place where I could share my news with the rest of the world. When they turned left on to the dual carriage way heading for Perth I have to say I was a little surprised as I thought that they may be taking me to a bigger city like Glasgow or Edinburgh to disclose my news to the world's media.

We headed into Perth and crossed the river Tay and headed up towards Kinnoull Hill and Murray Royal Hospital. I was now getting a little scared and when we turned into the hospital entrance I was even more scared but I just told myself that this was all part of some test that I would have to go through to prove what I was saying was true and also to prove I was not crazy. We pulled up in front of Moredun B which was the ward for male patients and I got out of the car and headed up the stairs to the ward. The first person I saw was a lady who was cleaning the stairs and I said to her "Christ the person who created the universe guided me here". She looked at me as if I was completely crazy and I think that she probably thought I was going to be in the ward for a very long time.

The first doctor I saw was Dr Peterson and he definitely didn't believe a word I was saying and prescribed Haloperidol. I have since learned that this drug should never be given to patients with Dystonia as it can cause a dystonic reaction. I assumed that Dr

Peterson was part of God's grand scheme and this was another test so as I asked him whether I should take the medication I winked at him but of course he had no idea why I was winking at him and he just thought this was another sign of my illness. Anyway even though I knew I did not need the medication I took it and when I went back to my bed I immediately had a dystonic reaction. This at the time was very confusing as I thought that I had done everything that God wanted yet I had still had this reaction but when the effects of the Haloperidol wore off I realised that I had not imagined any of this and I was still being guided by God.

That evening I went into a toilet cubicle to have a pee but unbeknown to me I was being observed by the staff very carefully. Now I have had a bashful bladder for as long as I can remember so it can take some time for me to urinate especially if there are nurses outside waiting for me. Anyway this particular time I could not go and as the nurses were demanding that I come out I thought I better do what they say. I started to walk along the corridor towards the locked front door of the ward with one nurse called Scott on one side of me and a much bigger nurse Luke on the other side. Now there was no premeditation in this but suddenly I started to bolt for the front door but the nurses must have sensed I was going to do this as before I got more than five steps Scott tripped me up and I went crashing down. Luke then pinned my right arm to the ground, but after I told him about my shoulder surgery he loosened his grip a little. Now as I was lying there pinned to the floor from the depths of my throat I cried out "Crawford" because I wanted them to realise that despite everything that had happened to me over the last three days I was still me and I was not claiming to be anyone else. It felt a bit like the film 'Braveheart' where William Wallace cries out 'Freedom'!

After a few minutes the nurses let me get back to my feet and I went to sit on a nearby seat. I was very calm but the on call doctor obviously didn't think so as the next thing I knew I am in the TV room and I'm surrounded by several nurses. I'm not stupid and I realise that they are not all there to wish me goodnight or certainly not verbally anyway. My assumption was correct and before I can do anything about it I was pinned to the floor and my jeans are taken down to allow one of the nurses to inject my backside with something which was supposed to knock me out. The thing is as I'm being pinned down this voice builds up inside me and I scream out "I'm Jesus Christ". The nurses let me go and I go back to my bed to sleep of the injection they have just given me. I have seen my notes relating to my admission and they make interesting reading. They claim that I was suffering from paranoia and auditory hallucinations. Now I can almost accept the paranoia as remember I thought God had let everybody else in on his grand scheme but obviously it was only me. As for the auditory hallucinations well I never have then or since heard voices of any kind and that is why my records say I deny this because it just isn't true. Despite my very strong religious beliefs I have always known that despite the fact that God guides me every day I am still Crawford Buchan and not any more special than the next man. I can't perform miracles or heal open wounds or take away the pain of losing a loved one. I'm just an ordinary man who has been given this incredible gift to know without doubt that God exists the only problem was I had absolutely no idea how I was going to prove it to the rest of the world. I was given an EEG and a CT scan but these were largely unremarkable. Despite my improvement over the three weeks since my admission to the hospital the next psychiatrist still decided that the best course of treatment for me was Lithium. My Mum was present at this consultation and she was not happy that I was basically being offered medication just because I wanted to help people all over the world. The psychiatrist at one point even said that I was being over familiar with people. Apparently this meant I was saying good morning to people I didn't even know. It seemed very strange that she actually thought that this was a bad thing! At one point my Mum even said that "Crawford was the sanest person in our family". I also did not want to start taking Lithium so I said to the psychiatrist" give me two days and I will prove to you that I don't need to start taking Lithium".

The next day I had two visitors. The first was Brian Bain our local minister and the second was James Simpson the former moderator of the Church of Scotland. I had now come to realise that I would be able to do a lot more good outside the hospital than inside it and when Brian and Jim came into my room I broke down in floods of tears. I couldn't understand how I could be locked up just because I believed in God. Brian and Jim were the first people that believed in me and I don't know to this day what Brian did behind the scenes to get me out but all I know is that at lunch time the next day he and I had some very tasty fish and chips in the staff canteen. I felt completely at ease with Brian because he was never going to judge me and even if he didn't believe that I could prove that God existed he certainly knew that I should not be locked up for believing in God. I was discharged the next day and therefore avoided a course of Lithium. It is strange to think that the reason I was locked up was that I believed in God and the reason I was allowed home was that they could not justify keeping me because I believed in God. Over the next few weeks I started to have certain doubts not only about my purpose in life but also in my faith. My religious feelings were not nearly as strong which meant my Dystonia was harder to deal with as I felt that I could not lean on God for support anymore. Also as I began to get more and more consumed by my Dystonia my mood came crashing down to that dark place I knew only too well. The only things keeping me going at that time were my trips down South to play the bagpipes on TV and as the pre-match entertainment at some lower league football games!

Brian Bain's son had a flat in Perth at South Inch Terrace which was just across the road from the prison in Perth and this was empty when I was discharged. Brian was willing to rent this flat out to me when I left hospital. It was quite a small flat on the fourth floor of the tenement with a kitchen/sitting room, bathroom and bedroom but it was ideal for me as I didn't really want to stay with my parents as I always wanted my independence. I was not working so I was grateful to the benefit system for keeping my head above water and putting food on my plate. Not having a daily routine of work meant that the days and weeks were quite long even with the piping appearances. I had managed to appear on some TV shows playing them as about the only thing I could play well was 'When the Saints go Marching In' which was my local football teams anthem. By doing a couple of phone ins I managed to get myself spots on Sky Sports 'Soccer AM' and channel fours 'Under the Moon' as well as the BBC's football program 'Offside'. I also volunteered my services for pre-match entertainment at Torquay United and Cambridge United as I had a crush on the female presenter from Soccer AM who was a Torquay fan. Unfortunately she was not wooed by my piping. I placed an advert in the St. Johnstone program about Dystonia to try and raise awareness.

The next gainful employment I had was for the BBC in Glasgow but it was not in front of the camera. They were implementing a new SAP accounting system and needed people to man the helpline in case their employees had any problems. I did this for three months staying with my brother Scott in Glasgow during the week and coming back to Perth at the weekends. I did not enjoy the job because I have to admit I didn't really know much about SAP. This must have gone unnoticed as I was offered an extension to my short term contract after three months. I decided to decline this as the whole family was heading off to Portugal for a two week holiday and I did not want to have to come back to this job. My mood when I returned from Portugal was very low and after seeing my local GP and admitting to frequent suicidal thoughts I was referred to another psychiatrist Dr Peterson who although in agreement with the GP that I had relapsed into a depressive state was slightly surprised that I appeared almost cheerful and matter of fact during appointments. I should point out I only knew of this medical history because I obtained a copy of it from my doctor after my last manic episode in 2008. On this occasion in November of 1999 I was not admitted but started on a course of medication which was changed some weeks later as there had been no improvement in my mood.

The next entry in my medical notes is for May 2000 where my neurologist thought that a course of Fluoxetine had caused a relapse in my symptoms of Dystonia although he did think that my general mood had stabilised. I was referred to clinical psychology but it was concluded that this would be of no benefit to me.

CHAPTER THREE

I had not worked since I gave up the job at the BBC and I think my Mum worried that I was becoming even more of a recluse. She had a chance meeting with Joe the man who used to be the golf professional at Craigie Hill golf club where I had been a member since I was twelve years old. He was opening a new golf centre in town and he asked me if I wanted to come and work there. I don't know if he actually needed someone to help him. It was just Joe being nice and it was a good opportunity to get out of the house each day. I really enjoyed working in the shop and this relaxed atmosphere meant that my Dystonia improved. Towards the end of 2002 I took a golf teaching course near Falkirk. It was a one week intensive course but by the end of it I was a qualified European Golf Teaching Federation coach although Joe called me a scab as he had got his qualification the hard way over three years!

As my neck was feeling better I thought I would make the most of the reprieve and I managed to get a job coaching golf for ten weeks at a kid's camp in up-state New York. It was at Kutcher's Sports Academy which was where I had spent a summer during university fourteen years before as a camp counsellor also teaching golf. I needed to bring a medical certificate to camp with me this time and as my brother-in-law Brian was American I asked him how the camp director would react to seeing in capital letters at the top of mine that I had manic depression. Although he didn't know the camp director my brother-in-law suggested if I wanted to keep my job at the camp that I may be better using a bottle of Tipex to hide this. Initially because I obviously didn't want to go all the way there just to be put on the next plane back I took Brian's advice and did Tipex out 'manic depression'. However after some more deliberation I decided that I should not be ashamed about my illness and also if anything happened to me it was important that my medical certificate was accurate.

I arrived in New York at the end of June 2003. I spent a night in one of the hostels in New York before catching the bus up to the camp the next day. Fortunately the hostel was not the YMCA which I had stayed in the last time I had gone to the camp in 1989 as believe me it does not live up to the song. It is not fun to stay at the YMCA! As a naïve nineteen year old boy on his first trip to the states in 1989 I found the constant sound of police sirens and the multitude of strange characters very scary. I felt a lot more confident on my second visit and I couldn't wait to get back to the camp where I had enjoyed such a great summer fourteen years ago.

The camp was just as I remembered it although when we arrived there were no children so it felt decidedly empty. The calm before the storm. As a coach my accommodation had moved up a notch. Instead of staying in a dorm with 12 eleven year olds to look after I now had a single room with en-suite facilities. It wasn't the Ritz but I knew how hard I had found it to get some peace and quiet during my first experience at the camp so having a space to call my own was a real step up.

The children who were between the ages of 8 and 18 started to arrive during the first weekend of July. The camp was a rich Jewish camp so as the children were dropped off by their parents a long queue of expensive vehicles snaked its way down the drive and out on to the road. We were responsible for helping to unload the massive trunks each child had packed for their four week stay. They could stay for eight weeks but it was usually just the four. Just enough to give their parent's a break from the responsibility of looking after them for a while. Believe me if you saw how some of these children behaved then you would know why the parents needed a break. Unfortunately we were not the ones who had spoilt the kids rotten or taught them that you didn't have to respect your elders or that basically they could get away with anything within reason. We were only the ones who would have to deal with the fallout from this lack of discipline.

Some of the coaching staff were the same as fourteen years ago. However I was still surprised to see that Joel the head golf coach was still in charge as he must have now been into his late seventies. However despite his increasing age his enthusiasm for golf and teaching it to the kids had not dwindled. Although certain facilities at the camp had been upgraded the golf practice area was not one of them. It was situated within a solid nine iron or an easy eight of the camp medical centre. Some of the golf coaches, apart from me, had been known to take a five iron down to lessons with them so that they could clear the medical centre and the road behind it but a lot of the time they only succeeded in breaking its windows. The practice mats were placed in a great big curve from the top of the hill to the bottom. I always thought that this could be a bit dangerous as a shank from a golfer on a top mat could feasibly hit someone at the bottom. There was also a small green with a couple of bunkers at the bottom of the hill to practice your short game. However this didn't get used very often as American's were only interested in how far they could hit it and not in their short game.

I used to like taking the kids down to the short game area because usually these were the children who knew a bit about the game and realised that the short game was the most important part. They were prepared to listen even if my own short game was lagging well behind that of even a scratch amateur.

I had been at the camp for about two weeks or ten days and I was really enjoying my new role as golf coach. I did not like staying on campus after dinner as I liked to get away from everything and relax with some friends in the bars of the nearest town Monticello. At this point in my life I had also not given up my smoking habit so at least when I was of campus I could do this without having to skulk of like a naughty schoolboy and hide behind the tennis courts. I enjoyed having a quiet beer, a smoke and a game of pool while meeting some of the locals. The camp ran one of the yellow school buses into town each night from the front gate at 9.00pm. It was a Wednesday night on July 6th. I'm not exactly sure of the date but it was in or around that day. I was at the front gate waiting on the bus to come up the hill from the gymnasium where it was always parked during the day.

As I waited I was talking to one of the other golf counsellors. As I was talking to him I saw Oksana one of the kitchen staff walking towards me. Oksana was a beautiful nineteen year old girl from Belarus. I didn't know her that well but we'd had a quick chat about nothing in particular in the camp foyer a few days ago. Now I have not always been good with names especially foreign ones so when she walked past me looking a bit down I said "smile Oskana". She turned her head and looked directly at me, even though her name was Oksana and I had pronounced it wrong, without breaking stride she smiled at me. It was the most beautiful smile I had ever seen and it was almost as if she floated past me in her goddess state.

I was still talking to the golf counsellor when there was an almighty bang which I can only describe as being like when you hold the lid of your wheelie bin fully open and let it fall shut. Over my friends left shoulder I saw Oksana's body being flung into the air. I knew it was Oksana because she had been dressed in or holding something red and as I saw her body in the air I thought for one sickening moment that this was the blood from her head hitting the windscreen! Her body must have travelled about thirty feet before it came down but by that time I had already gone into automatic pilot mode. I turned away from the front gate and started to run up the driveway to the main foyer screaming "call 999". I know now it should have been 911 but as I said I was not only in automatic pilot mode but in shock. I also shouted "keep the kids away from the front gate" because I did not want any small children to have to see the aftermath of the accident. I charged into the foyer and shouted at the lady behind the desk to call 999 but fortunately she had already called 911.

She must have realised that I was in shock as she kindly allowed me to go behind the reception desk and showed me through to a comfortable sofa outside the camp director's office. I collapsed on to the sofa and burst into tears. Momentarily I tried to stop the flow of tears as there were two campers using a computer in the next room and I didn't want to cry in front of them. I was joined by one of the other golf counsellors who could see how distressed I was and he asked if he could get me anything. I said I would like a coffee with a lot of sugar in it as I thought the sugar might be good for the shock. After sometime he arrived with a tray with biscuits and some very sweet coffee. I tried to drink the coffee but my hand was shaking so much that he had to get me a straw to stop me burning myself. As usual my sweet tooth got the better of me and I tried one of the biscuits but my hand was shacking so much I could not even take it from the packet properly. The other golf counsellor said "are you going to eat that or just juggle with it". I would normally have found that very funny but I was not really in the mood for jokes. I kept asking if she was still alive and was told she was but in my head I really didn't believe anybody could survive such an impact. Sometime later I was aware of the sound of a helicopter overhead and realised that Oksana must have been getting transferred to hospital in this.

I felt a bit better after the coffee and biscuits but I was still very shaky when I was informed that the police wanted to take a statement from me as I was about the only eye witness. I got up gingerly and the other counsellor and golf coach supported me as I walked back down the drive towards the front gate where a police car was sitting waiting for me. As I walked out of the front gate the picture of Oksana's body flying through the air flashed in front of my eyes and I suddenly felt my legs go from under me.

Fortunately the camp doctor had also been walking along side me and he caught me before I hit the ground. I can remember him standing over me asking if I suffered from any underlying conditions. I didn't know what would happen regarding my bipolar but I thought this was not the time to hold anything back. I told him about my manic depression that had been stable for five years and also what medications I was taking for it. I was taken up to the camp medical centre and came round lying in a bed in one of the side rooms. When I came round in this room I was in a very confused state. I could see the flashing lights of the police cars outside the window so I knew that Oksana's accident had unfortunately not been a bad dream but I couldn't remember the chain of events leading up to it. For some reason I started to think that I had been out drinking and in driving home drunk must have knocked down Oksana.

In the room alone with me now was Joel the head golf coach and I think he could tell that mentally I was on the edge of a very high cliff. He proceeded to tell me how he was at the airport waiting for his father's plane to arrive and he saw it crash land in a ball of flames his Dad perishing in the process. I do not know if this story is true but Joel didn't really have any reason to lie and I certainly believed him. I think he was just trying to say we can see horrible things but we can recover from them. Joel's pep talk had the desired affect and I went to the bathroom where I composed myself before going to speak to the police.

I walked down the camp drive to the waiting police car. I thought I would be sitting in the passenger seat but the police officer ushered me into the back seat which was a little unsettling. He asked me to describe what I had seen but I must have still been suffering from shock as my statement was full of inaccuracies. For some reason in my statement I said that Oksana had been thrown 150 feet down the road. Off course she had only been thrown about 30 feet and I imagine that because I was so far out with my initial description that the police were not going to pay much attention to my eye witness account. When I got home I did phone up the investigating officer to clear up the errors in my original statement but it seemed that the case had been closed and the incident written off as a tragic accident. When I got out of the police car they were just removing the car that had hit Oksana from the road and on the right hand side of the windscreen the glass was moulded inwards into the shape of a head. This was obviously where Oksana's head had hit the windscreen. I managed to stop myself from throwing up but only just.

That evening unsurprisingly I could not get any sleep as I was unable to get the picture of Oksana being hit by the car out of my head. For some reason I also felt that this wasn't just a straight forward accident although I had no way of ever proving this. As I knew I wasn't going to get any sleep I decided that I would walk down to the front gate and see if I could make any sense of what had actually happened. There was now a cold chill in the air and the haze that was hanging over the wet grass was creating a very eerie scene as I walked down to the gate. The overnight security guard got a real fright as I walked past him. In my pocket I had a roll of twenty five cent coins that I had got for change for the washing machine earlier in the day and I started to put these down on the road where the car skid marks were visible. As I was doing this I noticed that the police had left one of their rubber gloves behind which I picked up. They had also left one of Oksana's shoes behind. I was concerned that Oksana's colleagues who worked in the kitchen would see this on their way to breakfast so I picked this up to. The security guard had now figured out what I was trying to do even if I still think he thought I was a bit crazy for doing this in the middle of the night. I roped him into standing in the middle of the road in a position near to where I thought Oksana must have been when she was struck by the car while I went to the spot where I had been when the accident had happened. One of the things that was really bothering me was the fact that I didn't hear the sound of the cars breaks before Oksana was hit. Surely the first thing the driver would have done was slam on the breaks before impact not after. Apparently the people who had been in the car were an elderly couple and while this was only speculation there was some talk that they may have been temporarily blinded by an oncoming car. Now as with most of these accidents it is not long before the rumour mill is hard at work. On American roads there are usually the lines which mark the edge of the road and then an extra probably three feet of tarmac before you get to the grass. In my mind Oksana had been standing on the three feet of tarmac when she had been hit by the right hand side of the oncoming car. Now of course there was absolutely no way I could prove this and because I had witnessed the impact from the side I couldn't tell whether Oksana had actually stepped out on to the road. The only people who know that were the elderly couple and of course I was not going to be able to ask them.

The day after the accident I had not got any sleep the night before and I was sitting in the front foyer of the camp when one of the ladies who worked at the reception came in. She asked me if I wanted to go into Monticello for some breakfast. As I didn't want to be alone with my thoughts I said yes. We drove into Monticello and stopped off at one of those traditional American diners. We sat down in one of the booths and I ordered coffee with sausages and scrambled eggs. I love these diners where you order coffee and that means that you can basically drink as much as you want. The waitress constantly came round to fill up our mugs but considering I had not slept in twenty four hours it was probably not the smartest thing to be drinking. The food came and it was the usual ridiculous American portion that could have fed the five thousand without requiring much of a miracle. Needless to say I couldn't even finish half of it so we got a doggy bag to take back to camp for the other receptionist. After breakfast the lady that had kindly treated me to my breakfast said that she always had a brisk walk after her food and although I wanted to get back to camp to hear if there had been any news on Oksana I thought it would have been rude to say no to the walk and as she had the wheels I couldn't really refuse anyway. I can't tell you anything about what we chatted about during breakfast or our smart twenty minute walk as I have no recollection of it. I think she realised that I was still going through the hell of the previous night and therefore did all she could to divert my mind on to other things which was very nice of her.

We got back to camp and most of that morning was a blur to tell you the truth. As Oksana had been working in the kitchens at the camp the entire kitchen staff, apart from the cooks, were given the morning of and the coaches and counsellors were put to work in the kitchens and tasked with serving the kids their breakfast. Now most of the kids were not aware of what had happened last night so there were a few strange looks when they saw who was serving them but although there were a few wisecracks most of them knew not to try our patience this morning. We had the morning golf lessons as usual

41

but in the afternoon we didn't go to Kutcher's Country Club as usual but to another local course that the camp sometimes used.

I did not realise it fully at that time but I was already showing the early signs of a manic episode. I felt as if I was suddenly this great golfer capable of any shot. Unfortunately I was still Crawford Buchan and my first drive was pushed wildly into the trees and I started off with a double bogey six! I was playing with two campers who I don't think realised what sort of state of mind I was in. My golf over the first four holes was shocking although I did hit a good drive over the hill to the par four fifth. I was left with a straight forward wedge to the green which I dumped in the front bunker. I then proceeded to leave my next shot in the bunker. I swore at this pathetic effort making sure the kids could hear followed by spitting on the green, playing out of turn and standing in the line of one of the kids putts. They looked at me strangely at this point but when I got to the next tee and asked them what I had done wrong they thought I was referring to the duffed bunker shot and not all the displays off poor etiquette which is what I had wanted them to correct me on. I now felt as if I could suddenly hit the ball three hundred yards of the tee but my super powers had not been transferred to my swing and I hit it about two hundred and fifty up the middle of the par five which I bogeyed. We joined Joel the head golf coach on the next tee where I proceeded to miss the ball intentionally followed by a loud four letter expletive. Joel reminded me that I should not use this language in front of the kids. As usual Joel hit a couple of drives neither of which he was very happy with. Joel swung the club flat like a baseball player so I advised him to move his right foot back about six inches to enable him to swing round his legs and generate more power. He did this and he hit an absolute cracker. I think he was more surprised than I was at this success. When we got to the par three eighth as I was about to hit my tee shot I suddenly felt as if I was drunk and was

42

going to be sick. I staggered of to the side of the tee as I thought I was going to throw up in the bin. I realised that by now my antics were becoming more and more noticeable to my playing partners. I quickly hit my tee shot and was glad I managed to finish the nine holes without any more weird outbursts.

 I got the bus back to camp but by now the lack of sleep and mental scars from the previous night was starting to catch up with me. I phoned my girlfriend in Scotland to tell her what had happened and she was very sympathetic. She and I had always had a very good and open sex life and she had even sent me some erotic photographs via e-mail when I was at camp with various fantasies we hoped to act out when I got back. Now another symptom of a manic episode is that sexual inhibitions are removed so when I phoned her it did end up being a very sexually arousing call. When you are manic all your sensations and I mean all are magnified and it can almost feel as if the person is there with you. I retired to my room for a cold shower! That night I could not get to sleep again so I found myself walking back down to the front gate to the scene of the crash. We are told before we go to camp to bring little things that show which country we are from with us, as the children like these. On my first visit as a counsellor I brought over the Lion Rampant flag and also some small tartan Haggis or is that Haggi! One camper asked me what beer sign the flag was for! This time Mum had given me a small wooden cross with some tartan on it to hang on my door.

 I took the cross of the door and headed down to the front gate. It was a different security guard from the previous night but he was equally as surprised to see me in the middle of the night. I walked up along the camp fence until I was near the front door of the kitchen staffs accommodation and I placed the small cross at the bottom of the fence and said a little prayer for Oksana. I was now very aware that I was now not really in control of my own actions. I don't know if you are aware of the biblical story of the footprints in the sand. Basically a man is walking alone along the beach but when he turns to face the direction from where he has just come there are two sets of footprints in the sand. Now one of these sets of footprints is his and the other set represents those of the Lord walking alongside him. The story goes on to tell of how the man turns around again only to see one set of footprints. This is when the man needs the Lord the most and he asks the Lord how can you leave my side when I need you the most? The Lord replies by saying that you know only too well that especially during your darkest moment I will always be by your side. Ever since I was first hospitalised it is when I turn to see only one set of footprints that I feel the most scared as this is when I know that I have to carry out God's wishes no matter how hard these will be or how scary. Unlike the psychiatrists who said that I was hearing voices it was only that I was willing to give my life over to God and entrust it to him no matter what the consequences. That evening I could feel that I was going to have to entrust my life to God again. I can categorically say that the last thing I wanted to do at that moment was die but because of the great gifts that had been bestowed on me I was willing to sacrifice myself to prove that God existed. I wondered past the security guard, out of the front gate and on to the road. I thought that God obviously wanted me to sacrifice myself like Oksana. I was walking along the edge of the road just waiting for the impact of the car on my body. I was terrified and then suddenly I felt myself being thrown into the air and I assumed I had been hit by a car. I landed heavily in the grass but to my surprise I was not unconscious and I did not feel any pain. Standing over me was the security guard who had seen me in the road and bundled me off it into the safety of the undergrowth. He asked me what I was playing at but obviously I could not give him an answer that he would ever comprehend. I went back to my room where I lay on my bed but I did not get any sleep.

That Friday I was actually due to have a day off and go to Philadelphia to watch a baseball game with one of the other golf coaches but because of the week's events those plans were knocked on the head. That afternoon the whole camp was going to the movies and we were given the option of going to help with the supervision if we wanted. As I wanted to take my mind of things I jumped at the chance to do something. I think the movie was Finding Nemo but I could be wrong as I fell asleep for a couple of hours during it. When I came out of the film one of the group leaders gave me an envelope that had about thirty dollars in it. Apparently you got paid for volunteering to supervise at these of campus excursions. As we were in a shopping mall I went off to spend the money. I went into one of those giant sports stores where I bought a baseball and a Yankees t-shirt. I also bought an amusing golf hat that I was going to give to one of the other staff members. We got back to camp just before dinner but at least most of the day had now passed without me thinking too much about the accident. I saw the camp doctor that day and told him that I wanted to go and see Oksana in hospital but he did not think this was a great idea considering my Bipolar and also the fact that she was in such a critical condition and hooked up to so many machines. I managed to persuade him that I would be able to cope with her condition and it was decided that I could go and visit her tomorrow as her parents were coming over from Belarus as well and I hoped that I would at least get a chance to talk to them.

That evening the normal kitchen staff were back working but there was a special serving stand in the middle of the dining hall for desserts. As the counsellors and some of the campers came up to get there sweets I was getting them to sign the baseball that I had bought earlier as I planned to take this to Oksana tomorrow so she would know that everyone at the camp was thinking and praying for her. Some of the people realised why I was getting them to sign it while I just told the others it was for a special Scottish baseball game that was going to be held when I got back. After dinner I saw Jenny who was Oksana's friend in the foyer of the camp. Jenny felt really guilty about the accident because the reason Oksana was crossing the road was to go to a basketball match. Now Oksana at first had not wanted to go but finally she was convinced although she hadn't been too happy about it. I sat down beside Jenny. On the table in front of Jenny was two large paper cups of water. I took my leg and lifted it up before kicking one of the cups over so that water went everywhere. Jenny as you would expect looked at me as if I was crazy. I asked her if she wanted me to knock over the other cup of water and she nodded her head. I lifted my leg again and kicked over the second cup of water. A small smile started to appear on her face. I said to her that it had been my choice to kick over the cups of water just as it had been Oksana's choice to go to play basketball. Now nobody knows what is round the corner for any of us but what is absolutely certain is that Oksana's accident was in no way her fault. I think despite Jenny's poor English that she understood what I was trying to tell her. We hugged emotionally and I left her sitting there. There were quite a few people in the foyer and I can remember throwing the baseball back and forth with a few of them.

I was still however very restless and couldn't decide whether I should get the bus of camp and into town as usual. I walked down the drive with the intention of catching the bus. When I got to the front gate I again suddenly felt the fear building up in me as I felt God was calling on me again to prove that he existed by sacrificing myself. I walked out on to the road and lay face down on the tarmac. I could see the lights of an oncoming car in the distance. At that moment the same security guard who had bundled me off the road last night, along with another couple of counsellors who had no idea what I was doing, picked me up and escorted me off the road. The security guard was very concerned and wanted to tell somebody what I was trying to do but I begged him not too and managed to convince him that it would not happen again. I walked back up to the foyer off the camp deciding that it would probably be better if I didn't go off camp tonight. I had almost got to the foyer when I suddenly changed my mind and turned to walk back for the bus. The camp medical centre was on the right of the drive as you walked towards the main gate and as I got too it I suddenly felt drawn towards it. I walked up the steps opened the door and walked towards the reception desk. I had only taken a couple of steps when my legs went from under me but fortunately one of the medical team was at my side and they caught me before I crashed to the ground. I came round in a single bed. I was aware that there was a camper in a single bed across from me but I had no idea what was wrong with him and at that point I didn't really care as I was mentally fried. I can remember shouting at the top of my voice "I'm Tiger Woods". Not surprisingly it wasn't long before an ambulance arrived to take me to hospital. I was moved on to the wheeled trolley and handcuffed to it. There was also a metal bar positioned tightly across my legs. It was only when I was in the ambulance and I saw my reflection in the window that reality set in. The camp doctor was in the ambulance with me. I held my hand out in front of my face and said to him that I was obviously the wrong colour to be Tiger Woods. He smiled in agreement. I asked him if he could loosen the metal bar that was digging into my shins and as he now realised that I was no longer a threat he did this as quickly as he could, almost apologetically. As I had now lost all notion of time I'm not sure when I arrived at the Monticello Medical Centre which was the nearest hospital.

CHAPTER FOUR

For some reason the only real memory of my initial admission to the hospital was feeling extremely cold and having to ask for another blanket. I can't remember even seeing a doctor before I was eventually moved to the psychiatric ward. As I was going to the ward I took of my caterpillar boots. Paul the other golf coach didn't know why I had done this. I knew I would not be allowed the laces on the ward so I thought I would save them the bother of confiscating them. I was terrified going into the psychiatric unit as even though I had been sectioned in Perth I didn't know what to expect in America. The nurse that took my details when I arrived did not fill me with confidence as he was having difficulty understanding my accent. I gave him the contact numbers of my next of kin but I asked him not to phone my Mum or Dad as I didn't want to worry them. I was shown to my room which was nothing special but I was the only one in it and there was en-suite facilities. The full realisation of my predicament began to sink in. I was three thousand miles from home locked up in an American psychiatric unit without a change of clothes or a cent in my pocket. I had been booked into the facility in the middle of the night so it was not until the next morning that I met any of the other patients or nursing staff. There were a few strange characters to say the least, from one who looked like a night club bouncer to a traditional Jewish man. I tried to keep myself to myself at breakfast until I was asked to fill in my menu for the next few days. At least this was the same procedure as in the psychiatric ward in Perth even if the food options were not. I decided to ask the American man mountain, who looked like a night club bouncer, what he would recommend and when he said the chicken I couldn't exactly disagree so I ticked it of for my evening meal. The funny thing was that due to my manic episode I was a little paranoid so when the chicken arrived that evening and tasted disgusting I jumped to the conclusion that he was trying to poison me! I saw the psychiatrist that afternoon and was about to tell him about all my religious feelings when he cut me down before I got started, rather like a strict school teacher, by saying "sit down Mr Buchan". The authority in his voice was just what I needed so I sat down. He explained to me that he felt that the manic episode had obviously been brought on by witnessing Oksana's accident but he felt that by increasing my medication it would not be long before my bipolar illness had stabilised again and I could go home.

I was visited that afternoon by Mr Black the camp director. I was still in the middle of my manic episode and I can remember singing to him "who wants to be a millionaire, I don't". This was a vague attempt to point out that I would not hold Mr Black responsible for the fact that he had not asked for my medical certificate when I arrived at the camp. If he had done he would have seen right at the top in capital letters that I had written "manic depression". When Mr Black agreed to take me on for the summer he had said that I would require a medical certificate which I had obtained. The reason he did not have it was he hadn't actually asked me for it since I had arrived at the camp. I was not trying to hide my medical condition from him as I'm not ashamed to admit I have a mental illness and but for the trauma of witnessing Oksana's accident then my mental state would have remained stable as confirmed by my psychiatrist before I left Scotland.

I think Mr Black realised that he should have asked me for my medical certificate as the next day he came to the ward with Joel and accused me of keeping things from them. He gave me a letter of dismissal saying I had not provided them with a medical history. Probably more surprising was the fact that Mr Black also wrote that it had been brought to his attention that I had not been taking my medication since shortly after arriving at the camp. This statement was completely untrue as I always took my medication and had done so since arriving at the camp. Mr Black also passed this unfounded information about my medication on to the Bunac representative because when she phoned up to apparently enquire about my health she said that she had heard I was not taking my medication! This was very distressing as she was obviously taking Mr Black's version of events to be the truth and the fact that there was absolutely no evidence that I hadn't been taking my medication didn't seem to matter. Obviously I was the one who was mentally ill so who would you believe. Joel and Paul the assistant golf coach came into visit me most days. I can remember one day where Joel was trying to show me how baseball players catch the ball near the wall before it goes for a home run. We were in the dining area and he was jumping into the metal lockers with his left shoulder to demonstrate this. Now I can't tell you if it was because of watching this or because I was again just following the footprints laid out for me by God. I'm sure it was the latter but that evening I was taking a shower when I suddenly felt this great pull towards the main door. The next thing I knew I was stark naked and running down the corridor towards the front door. As my feet were wet it was hard for me to get any grip on the linoleum floor and I must have resembled Bambi on ice, apart from the cute bit! I got up to stop speed and proceeded to charge head first into the locked metal door. As I did this I turned my body just as Joel had been showing me during his baseball lesson earlier so it was my left shoulder that took most of the impact. I rebounded off the door and ended in a crumpled heap on the floor. Nurses soon appeared with a blanket and I was escorted back to my room. I was now standing in front of my mirror the adrenalin still rushing through my blood. I felt invincible and I banged my mouth of the metal shelf below the mirror as if to prove that I felt no pain. About half an hour later one of the nurses came to get me and as we were standing in the corridor he told me that I would be going for a CT scan to make sure I had not damaged my head when I collided with the main door which I had apparently managed to break. I looked at him and asked if he wanted me to start from ten yards further back this time! He looked at me to check whether I was being serious and we both laughed.

The CT scan was clear and the door had obviously come of a lot worse than me as it had to be replaced. I went back to the ward to try and settle down. I tried to occupy my mind by doing a jigsaw and also participating in some of the therapy offered. This did work for a short time but when the medication was due just before we retired for the night I could feel me becoming more and more agitated. I took the pills and threw them across the dining hall explaining that it was my choice to refuse the medication. It felt a bit like that first time in Murray Royal where I was tackled to the ground by the nurses so I decided that I would do things under my own terms this time. I went back to my room and asked the nursing staff to tie me to the bed with restraints. Now although the nurses will not do this in the UK they do it in America so at my own bequest I was tied to the bed using leather arm and leg restraints. One of the nurses who I had got to know and really liked was sitting in my room across from me and he said "Why are you doing this Crawford"? I looked him straight in the eyes and said that I was doing it to prove that God existed. He seemed to think that this was an impossible task and so he asked me how I proposed to do this. Even though I did not want to die I told him that I was willing to sacrifice myself to prove that God existed. Just as I said this my body began to be thrown about the bed like a rag doll. It felt as if I was re-enacting my car crash in 1997. Several more nurses entered my room followed by the on call doctor. I explained to the doctor that I did not blame her for anything that was about to happen to me as a result of her treatment. In my head this was where I was going to die and I therefore thought that the medication that she was going to give me was going to kill me. I was held down by the nurses and injected three times in my backside. Despite four or so nurses holding me down I felt the same voice building up inside me that had cried out in similar circumstances in Murray Royal Hospital in 1998. Now I want to make it clear that I no point then or since have I heard voices contrary to the opinion of several psychiatrists. "I'm Jesus Christ" I screamed and then I burst out laughing saying "no I'm not I'm Crawford Buchan". What I'm trying to say is that I have been given this wonderful gift to prove God exists and also that he walks among us today and every day. After the injections had started to take hold of my system I began to question whether I had done the right thing. Every bone in my body started to ache and I curled myself up into a small ball. I was so thirsty and the nurse who had questioned my reasons for doing this in the first place gave me a drink of Pepsi through a straw with a look on his face that said, I told you this was going to happen but you didn't listen.

I closed my eyes and I do not know what happened over the next few hours but I woke to find myself in an entirely different room and in a different area of the hospital altogether. My chest was hooked up to a cardiac monitor for some reason. To this day I have no idea how or why I got to be in that position but all I can say for definite is that I was now feeling much better than when I had closed my eyes in the ward hours earlier. I don't know this for certain but it seems that after I had received my three injections the nurse was still monitoring my blood pressure and it appears that this may have fallen dangerously low so I was transferred to the intensive care unit to be monitored. These details could only be confirmed as fact by the hospital records but what's certain is that I had again put my life in God's hands and he had protected me. This overwhelming feeling of love meant that I wasn't really curious about the sequence of events that had taken place that night.

After spending a few more hours hooked up to the heart machine I was given the all clear to be transferred back to the psychiatric ward. I now felt a great empathy for my fellow patients and wanted to help them. Unfortunately I was unable to help Herman the Jewish man because his family thought he would get better treatment in a private facility and so the last time I saw him he was being wheeled out of the ward on a trolley. Unfortunately his family thought that if you threw enough money at a mental illness then it could be cured. Herman's surroundings were not going to improve his condition and I often wonder what became of him.

There was also a young girl on the ward who admitted to me that she had hit her teacher. Unfortunately she thought this was a cool way to behave but I think that I managed to get her to realise that what she had done was wrong. A few of the other patients were drug addicts who had chosen the psychiatric ward for treatment instead of having to start a prison sentence. There was one very old lady who I think most of the staff had just given up on. One evening she was sitting at the other end of the dining table. I had now got most of my possessions brought over from the camp. I say most because I was to find out later that several of my US dollar traveller's cheques had gone missing when my room was cleared out. I now had the baseball that I was going to give Oksana back so I proceeded to roll this across the dining table to her. I think the nursing staff were surprised to see her stop it with one hand and roll it back to me with the other. We carried on doing this for a few minutes until my visitors arrived. I felt sorry for her as the nursing staff explained to her that I was going back to Scotland soon and she became visibly upset saying that all the good people in her life always left her.

CHAPTER FIVE

I had booked my flight back to Scotland on the internet so when I got the all clear from the doctor I said my goodbyes and caught the bus to New York. As I was waiting for my flight to be called for boarding my name was called out over the tannoy and my presence was requested at the boarding desk. To my surprise I had been upgraded to first class for the first time in my life. I took my luxurious leather seat in first class with enough leg room for me to stretch out fully. The pilot then announced that if somebody gave up their seat they could spend the night in a hotel in New York and have the extra bonus of $500 spending money. As I thought this would be the only time I travelled first class I was not going to give up my seat unless it was a matter of life and death. The flight back was very relaxing and I even managed to get ice cream with toffee sauce before I landed! My sweet tooth has always been my weak point. The day after I arrived back I went straight back to work at the golf centre.

Joe was delighted to see me back but was obviously concerned about my state of mind. I saw Dr Burnell at Murray Royal and he offered me counselling but I declined this offer and did as I always did and dealt with things on my own although as usual after a manic episode I still felt that God was watching over me. Unfortunately this feeling of well-being usually only lasted a few months before my mood nosedived back into depression. I was very happy to see my girlfriend again as she understood my illness and what I was going through. I can't speak for her but sex was even better than before I left. She was a free spirit and it is really only now that I wish I had done more to hang on to her but at that time I was unable to feel love. I could try and contact her now through a mutual friend but I think that boat has sailed even if I would still jump at the chance of having a normal date with her and taking it from there.

She worked at the time for a small advertising firm who would produce brochures and literature for other small companies. I had written a poem for Oksana's mum who I had seriously considered going to see in Belarus. My girlfriend got the poem printed in some special covers which looked like they had Angels on them. I thought that Oksana's mother might like to know that the last thing Oksana did was smile but after getting in contact with her through Oksana's friend Jenny I realised that she thought that Oksana had slowed to speak to me and this in some way may have contributed to her death. I obviously knew that this was not the case but even to this day Oksana's death troubles me the most because it feels as if she died to teach me another lesson from God in the psychiatric ward in America. I also realise that there was a reason I was not killed in my suicide attempt in 1997 and that I have to do as much as I possibly can now to prove that God exists. The poem I wrote was simply called "Smile Oksana".

The lips make the gesture,
Body oblivious to the adventure.
He seems to play a mysterious game,
She never felt the pain.

As she smiled at me from afar,
Her destiny was already a floating star.
As she watches over all of us,
Wondering why there's all the fuss.

When our children are far away,
We can't watch over them every day.
As he decides what will be done,
Even when the pain's hard to overcome.

Oksana is now in a better place,
Her graceful walk and pretty face,
You will join her in a while,
And Once again see her Angelic smile.

I continued to work in the golf centre until the end of 2006 when due to rent increases Joe decided that now was a good time to close. Apart from my depression caused by my bipolar and chronic pain associated with my Spasmodic Torticollis my mood had remained reasonably stable for eighteen months. I had not done any work since the golf centre closed at the end of 2006 when Olav a very good Norwegian friend who ran a company (Broxwood Scotland Ltd) importing windows and doors from Norway phoned me up and asked if I wanted to help out in the office on an unpaid basis. Although at first I was a bit unsure about this I decided I had to do something to get me out of the house. The position only involved sending out brochures and letters to prospective clients so it was not in the least bit stressful and the staff at Broxwood were very nice and made me feel part of the team. I had been doing this for about eight months when at the start of 2007 I was offered the opportunity to become part of the paid workforce which I jumped at as I was now able to earn my own money and it gave me back some of my independence. I didn't have to rely on hand outs anymore and could pay my own bills and even afford to run my small Peugeot to and from work. Even though the work was not stressful my neck was getting worse and by April 2008 I was finding it harder and harder to get a good night's sleep.

Then after two sleepless nights I awoke one Thursday morning to find that the pain in my neck had completely disappeared. Now even though I was delighted by this sudden change I was also very sceptical about the cause. I always say that nobody really knows you as well as you know yourself and this certainly applies to me and my mental state. I was concerned that this sudden improvement in my Dystonia could be put down to my lack of sleep and also the early signs of another manic episode. I decided to phone Murray Royal Hospital and seek help. Unfortunately it was just after 5.30pm when I phoned and so there was only a junior doctor available. She didn't seem that concerned about my mental state and when I asked to speak to one of her more senior colleagues she proceeded to record in my notes that I had been rude on the phone. Now I can assure you that I was not at all rude. I just wanted to speak to a doctor who would be best placed to diagnose a manic episode if indeed that was what I was about to have. As it was after hours the junior doctor informed me that I would have to call NHS 24 but she was unable to provide me with their number. That night I couldn't get to sleep again so I called NHS 24. I explained my situation and gave them a brief medical history and I was told that a psychiatric nurse would call me back as soon as possible.

I was called back fairly quickly and spoke to a very nice psychiatric nurse. I explained everything for a second time but the nurse said he was not concerned about my mental state. Unfortunately even when I'm having a manic episode I can carry on a perfectly normal conversation without my speech being pressured. However the nurse did say that he would fax my psychiatrist as a matter of urgency to get one of his staff to phone me the next day. On Friday I went to work as normal and even though I was probably a bit happier than usual my elevated mood was not noticed by any of my colleagues. I work from ten in the morning until 2.30pm so I got home around about three in the afternoon. There were no messages on the answering machine. You may wonder why I didn't just phone my psychiatric team myself. Unfortunately at that time in my life I didn't have a very good grasp on my illness and the best ways to stay well. It was still very difficult for me to ask anyone for help.

5.30pm came and went so I realised that either the nurse from last night had not sent the fax or the psychiatric team in Perth hadn't got it. In my head I had the picture of this fax with my name on it being hidden in amongst other papers. This would have been almost acceptable but the real reason was that my psychiatrist had got the fax but he and his team had been too busy to phone me that Friday. That night I couldn't get to sleep so I phoned NHS 24 again. I went through the same procedure as the night before and again the psychiatric nurse seemed to think I wasn't having a manic episode because my speech was still not pressured. The next day I phoned my brother. I was crying because I thought I was definitely going back to Murray Royal. Scott was also upset but he tried to reassure me that everything would be fine. That night the lack of sleep was now having a serious effect on my mood. I phoned Carl my best mate who lives in Australia and we were on the phone for a long time and I started to get the strong religious feelings again where I was going to have to sacrifice myself to prove that God exists. I had the thought that I was going to hang myself on the back of my bedroom door. I didn't want to die so I picked up the phone and phoned my Mum to tell her what I didn't want to do but I felt I had to do. She told me that Dad was driving down as we spoke. For what seemed like an age before Dad arrived Mum talked to me on the phone and managed to talk me out of hanging myself. When Dad arrived he didn't even ask me how I was feeling. This was just another crazy outburst from his youngest son. I was also surprised that he was also fully dressed. If my son had phoned to say he was about to hang himself then I think I would have made do with a dressing gown and a heavy foot on the accelerator! He drove me back up to their house in Clathy where I tried to get some more sleep. I had Harvey the dog for company but I probably only slept for an hour at most.

Now on the Sunday my football team St.Johnstone were playing Rangers in the semi-final of the Scottish Cup and I was supposed to be going with my brother and Dad. I managed to persuade Dad and Mum that I was well enough to go to the game. Mum drove us down to my brothers as he lived about a twenty minute walk away from the stadium where the game was taking place. Now shortly after I had been admitted to Murray Royal hospital for the first time in 1998 I had started playing my bagpipes at the St Johnstone games which had led to a few TV appearances and one radio show. On the Saturday before this semi I had phoned the Sunday Post newspaper to say that I may bring my pipes to the game but I would only play them if we were winning. I know that Dad didn't want me to take them to the game but I managed to take them down in the car with me by saying that I was only going to play them in Scott's garden.

I did play them in the garden before the game but unbeknown to my Dad I also phoned the head of security at Hampden Park to make sure it would be ok to play them at the game. He said it was, so as I could not set off with my pipe box, I slipped my chanter into my inside jacket pocket and headed off to the match with Scott, James his son and Dad. As we were going to the game I went into a newsagents and bought a Sunday Post. I had a quick flick through it and was surprised to find that there was indeed an article on the possible return of the Saints piper. I showed this to James who quickly realised that the article was about me. When we got to the stadium I let Dad go in first as I finished my cigarette and then found a steward. I showed the steward the chanter as I had been instructed to do by the head of security and I was allowed in without any problems. I took my seat in the stands next to this very nice girl. I remember as the game started that there were a lot of balloons on the pitch and we were joking together that these might interfere with the game as the wind blew them from side to side. I showed her the newspaper article and then opened my jacket a bit like a flasher to show her the chanter. Now Rangers were by far the better team in the first half but the game was still goalless at half-time. This filled me with hope as I knew we couldn't be as bad in the second half. My optimism was not unfounded as we did much better in the second half and we were close to forcing the game into extra-time. I had decided that it was a good time to get the chanter out and play 'when the saints go marching in'. Unfortunately my Dad didn't share this view as the minute he saw the chanter his face contorted with rage. Now I was a 38 year old man so surely it was up to me if I played or not and I had also got permission to do so from the security staff at the game.

Anyway because of his reaction I got up and left my seat. I walked down to the concessions area underneath the stand where you could buy pies and drinks. This area was deserted now apart from the odd staff member tidying up behind the counters. I took out my chanter and started to play. I think the remaining staff behind the counters must have got a fright as the pipes were so loud under the low ceiling of the stand above. I decided that I was going to play for the fans and the team despite what my Dad had said. I went up to a police officer who was standing just at the entrance to the stand. I checked with him that it was ok for me to play and when he gave me the go ahead I headed out towards the open air of the stand. This felt like my tunnel on to the hallowed turf of Hampden Park. As I emerged I felt something wet land on my face and I realised that I had been spat on by the Saints supporters in the row above. Now I have always despised spitting so it was hardly surprising that I reacted very angrily to this but in doing so I forgot the police man was still standing beside me. He grabbed me before I had a chance to react and pulled me back under the stand. Just as this was happening the final whistle had been blown and fans started to stream out for a comfort break before the start of extra-time. The police man reminded me that I would be the one arrested if I reacted. I was so disgusted that I was seriously considering leaving the stadium and walking back to my brother's house. However I decided that I wanted to face up to the fans that had spat on me so I made my way back to my seat but on the way I gave those fans sitting in the front row a dose of the worst evil stare I could muster. I sat back down in my seat but I was no longer watching the game as I was texting my mates to tell them what had just happened to me. As a result I missed St. Johnstone taking the lead with a header in the first period of extra-time. I didn't even stand up to celebrate which the people next to me obviously found strange. I think my Dad half turned to hug me but I was still sitting texting and the girl on my right also looked down strangely wondering why I had not reacted.

I had now lost all interest in the football and was more interested in my mobile phone. I decided I was going to leave so I stood up and thanked the girl next to me for her company. I don't think she could believe that I was going to leave with my team leading 1-0 and only ten minutes to go. I left the stadium through a side entrance and as I did I was stopped by someone wanting to interview me for a subject that I have no recollection of now. As I walked around the stadium there was some youngsters sitting on the main steps to the Hampden entrance so I gave them a quick burst of 'When the Saints go Marching in'. I then came across two police officers. I asked them what would happen if I continued to play my chanter and they advised me that I would be arrested for a breach of the peace. This surprised me as when a friend, my brother and I had been walking to the game there were a couple of pipers busking. My friend pointed out that they were playing 'Bonnie Dundee' as he was a Dundee supporter who are our local rivals. As I was talking to the police officers my Dad rushed up behind me fearing that I was going to talk myself into trouble. As usual he had assumed the worst before actually asking me what I was saying to them.

We walked round to the corner where we had agreed to meet Scott and James after the game. I now knew via text that Rangers had equalised with a penalty in the second period of extra-time and that the game itself was going to penalties. I now also knew that it was difficult to keep up with a penalty shootout with texts so I only really knew what the outcome of the game was when Scott's final text confirmed we had lost on penalties. There was not a lot of conversation on the way back to Scott's although I was not really that down about the game probably because I was now on the verge of another manic episode. We didn't spend much more time at Scott's as Dad seemed very keen to get back to Clathy to take Harvey the dog out. During the journey back I had already decided that I didn't want to spend another night at Mum and Dad's so when we got back I was going to take Mum's car and head back to my flat. Unfortunately Mum did not agree with this plan even when I said that if she was concerned about my mental state she could drive me into my flat and spend the night with me. I was not at all happy about not getting my own way so I decided to call a friend. Mum reluctantly gave me the phone and I knew she was outside my bedroom door when I made the call as I could hear her intake of breath as I spoke to Olav, my boss and named person. I told Olav that my parents were refusing me medical attention and I needed help. Olav was a little surprised I think but he didn't ask any questions and said he would be there in fifteen minutes. I had already packed a few things into a bag but I wanted Mum to give me the small white Bible that had fallen open to Matthew chapter 25 all those years ago in 1998. I think as a stalling tactic Mum said she didn't know where it was but I wouldn't believe that she could misplace something so important to me and my language reflected the fact that I was not happy that she had apparently lost it.

I took the bag that I had put a few things in and my bagpipes case and set of down the drive. I got as far as the red telephone box in the village and sat down on my pipe case to wait for Olav. I think Mum took her car and drove down to the end of the road to get Dad who had already left to walk Harvey. Olav arrived about fifteen minutes later and gave me a big smile and asked if I was ok. I said yes and gave him a quick rundown of the day's events and the fact that I wanted a lift back to my flat in Perth. He said that would not be a problem but maybe we should go and have a word with my Mum first. I was a bit reluctant to do this but for my Mums sake I agreed. When we got to the house though I said that I would prefer to stay in the car. Olav went into the house and had a lengthy conversation with my parents. He then came out of the house with the phone and explained that Manny a good friend from university was on the other end of the line. I spoke to Manny for a few minutes as he tried to convince me to go back inside the house and speak to my parents. As he did not know any of the circumstances I didn't really pay much attention to what he was saying but eventually I did go back into the house.

We were all in the kitchen and I could see from the expression on Dad's face that he was raging. I have to say that I didn't help by encouraging him to have a go at me. The fact that I had said this all in front of Olav was only pouring flames on to the fire burning inside him. It was agreed that Olav would give me a lift back to my flat.

Olav came in for a coffee and a chat before he went back to his own house. It was quite late when Olav left the flat and although my mood must have appeared completely stable I was already very ill. I phoned my best friend Carl in Australia and must have been on the phone to him for a long time. I was still unable to get any sleep so I phoned NHS 24 again. This time they put me through to an organisation called 'Breathing Space'. I spoke to a nice young lady and explained my medical history and the problems I was having getting to sleep but I don't think she was experienced enough to give me the correct advice as she advised me to drink a cup of warm milk. Now at the time this seemed like a good idea so I did actually make myself a mug of warm milk but off course it didn't help me get to sleep. As I was lying in my bed I again suddenly felt that I couldn't control my own actions. I screamed for help from the couple downstairs and then went through to the sitting room where I phoned myself an ambulance. I grabbed my bag and my pipe box and went down to the front door. I had to get out of the flat but I had left the keys upstairs. Instead of getting the keys I decided to break the door down with my shoulder! Now this was not just a few weak shoulder charges into the glass door but fourteen stone thrown as hard as I could into it. Fortunately the door held as it would have been very nasty if it had given way and ended up on the concrete steps below. My downstairs neighbours were now outside my door trying to calm me down but this only really happened when I saw the flashing lights of the ambulance and police.

I was talked into getting the keys and opening the front door. I was greeted by two police officers who saw me lying at the bottom of the stairs. I tried to explain that I hadn't slept for seventy two hours and I had bipolar disorder. I was escorted barefoot with my bag and bagpipes into the ambulance. They accepted my explanation that I had packed the bag because I knew that I was going to 'Murray

Royal Hospital'. Now I only live two hundred yards from the accident and emergency department so it was not a long drive! I was shown on to a bed in the accident and emergency department and told that a doctor would be along soon. One of the nurses turned out to be a relative of a work colleague so I think I got some extra special treatment from her anyway.

I should point out at this time that when I'm having a manic episode and I experience my strong religious beliefs I assume that God has somehow informed everyone that I meet that I have been put on Earth to prove that he exists. It would be a lot easier if this was the case but unfortunately I now know only too well that this is not the case. I was experiencing all the symptoms now of a full blown manic episode with sexual inhibition and for some reason I also believed that Tiger Woods would be by my bedside when I opened my eyes as he would want to meet the one person on Earth who could categorically prove that God existed. Obviously this didn't happen but I did have a chat with the patient in the next bed to me about Craigie Hill where I played my golf. I was also very aggressive to one of the nurses who I had overheard making an inappropriate comment. I got out of bed and shouted in her face giving her one hell of a fright. The staff were very good but as expected I was shuffled into another ambulance to transfer me to Murray Royal Hospital. It turned out that one of the ambulance crew knew me from Secondary School but I was not really in a fit state to recognise him.

CHAPTER SIX

I climbed the stairs to ward Moredun B, where I had been in 1998. I still had my pipes and the bag of items I had quickly packed before leaving home in Clathy some hours ago. I was shown into one of the side rooms by one of the nurses who had first treated me in 1998. I was then assessed by a young second year psychiatrist of Chinese orientation. I just assumed that my behaviour in the accident and emergency department at Perth Royal Infirmary from where I had just been transferred had been relayed to this doctor and that I was about to be sectioned under the mental health act. However the young doctor seemed to be more interested in finding out why I had a set of bagpipes with me than finding out about my mental state. I just said that I had played the pipes at the hospital the last time I had been admitted in 1998 and so that is why I had brought them this time.

To my astonishment he accepted this explanation and said I could go. Even though it was now the early hours of the morning I phoned Olav, and asked if I could come round to his and he said that was ok. I left the hospital in my bare feet and got a taxi to Olav's. He then gave me a lift back to my flat with a quick stop off at Perth Royal Infirmary so I could apologise to the nurse I had shouted at before. I think she was very surprised to see me again so quickly as, like me, she expected I would have been admitted to Murray Royal.

As soon as I got back into my flat I grabbed my car keys and headed for Clathy. Each manic episode I have had since 1998 has been so similar yet so different and this one seemed to be the best and yet the worst since I was first diagnosed. It was the ultimate battle of good against evil and yet at times I was unable to tell the difference between the two. I wanted to live so badly but I was prepared to die to prove God existed. This may seem crazy to the sane but to the mentally ill it is completely logical and yet terrifying at the same time.

I was driving to my parent's house in what can only be described as a terror filled manic episode yet I was aware of everything around me in a clarity that belied the fact that I had only slept for three of the last seventy two hours. The whites of my knuckles were visible as I clenched the steering wheel so tight fearing that evil may win the battle and I would flip my car as I had done in 1997.

Somehow I managed to navigate the narrow lanes and I found myself back at my parent's house. I entered the house as if none of the previous seventy two hours had ever taken place and that I was the only one that had an inkling of sanity left. My parents were waiting anxiously at the door but I didn't stop as I made my way to my old room. At first I was going to have a shower despite the fact that it was now five in the morning but I changed my mind and came out of the bathroom and went back to my room. I now felt that although I still knew exactly what I was doing that I couldn't or simply didn't want to stop what was going to happen next.

I made my way up the stairs to my parent's room to find my father standing next to the bed in his dressing gown. I walked purposefully towards him and proceeded to grab his dressing gown lapels. I felt the strength cursing through my body as I lifted him of his feet and threw him on to the bed. Looking straight into his eyes and to the bottom of his soul I said "Don't you fucking ever put me down again because I have God by my side now". If he had believed in God, which I don't think he did, then the fear of God had just been put into him but only time would tell! As I left the bedroom he had already picked up the phone to call for help. I had assumed that he was calling the police but I have subsequently found out from my Mum that he was phoning to get medical assistance for me.

I walked out of the house with the old bag I had stuffed with things collected when I was growing up and my bagpipes. I stopped in the drive to smash my pipe box of the window of my Dads Audi but amazingly the window did not break. I know it sounds hard to believe but I now felt that I was back in control of what I was doing and more importantly I knew why I was doing these things. I marched to the end of the drive and pulled the green wheelie bins across the drive, took my coat off, took my chanter out and started playing 'When the Saints go Marching in". I continued up the road playing sporadically only to be passed by a local neighbour who stopped briefly in his car but when I told him that he shouldn't worry and the police had been called he carried on up the road. I stopped at the red telephone box in the village and dialled 999. I had thought when my Dad picked up the phone he was calling the police so I thought I better phone them to explain why I had assaulted him. I told them about the years of psychological abuse I had endured. My mum by this time had caught me up and was outside the phone box pleading with me to come back to the house. I think she took the receiver from me, as I left the phone box, to talk to the officer I had been speaking to. I carried on up the road playing my chanter stopping once to lie in the wet grass in front of a neighbour's house in a position of surrender in case the police arrived. I then continued up the road and out of the village but I was now worried that I may be shot by the police however crazy that seems so I stripped until I was completely naked so they could see clearly that I wasn't carrying a weapon! I saw the small police van approaching and I held out my arms holding only my pipe chanter with the Saints scarf I had bought earlier at the game tied to it. I fell to the ground as the officers got out of the van and I finally felt that after thirty eight years I was now safe.

The officers helped me to my feet and I was bundled into the small cage at the back of the van. The cage gave of a pungent smell of fresh urine and other bodily odours but I was more concerned that the van was now heading back towards my father who was further up the road. I was screaming "keep him away from me". The van stopped and the officer had a quick word with my Dad. The van then turned at the end of the road and started to head back into Perth. It was very noisy in the cage at the back of the van so it was impossible for me to have a conversation with either officer. I think one of them was called Mr Black but he may have given me a false name. I was slightly surprised when I realised that they were driving me to Murray Royal Hospital as I had just assumed I would be taken to the police station and charged with assaulting my father. When I arrived at the hospital one of the nurses came down to meet me while the officers got me to put my trousers back on to cover myself up.

I was admitted to the ward and the first person that attempted to see me was the junior psychiatrist who had failed to admit me about two hours before. I made it clear that I didn't want to see him as I had now lost all confidence in him. The first psychiatrist I saw was Dr Pretorius who prescribed various medications for me. At times the nurses had to hold me down to get me to take my medication and even then I tried to regurgitate them. Now as with my other manic episodes I had some very strong religious beliefs but even so I still at all times knew that I was Crawford Buchan and therefore I unfortunately did not possess any super powers!

I can't remember too much about the first few days in the ward as the episode had gone untreated for three days since the initial symptoms and therefore my mental state had deteriorated quickly. According to my medical notes I assaulted a nurse on the ward which I have no recollection off. I find this very hard to accept as although I'm usually verbally aggressive when I have an episode I have never actually raised an arm to any of the medical staff treating me. I have tried to find out more about this assault if only to apologise to the nurse involved but I have been unable to establish the exact details. As my mood did not improve over the first few days using anti-psychotic medication it was deemed necessary for me to be transferred to the IPCU unit at Carse View in Dundee. I can't even remember the journey to this unit and I have absolutely no recollection of my two weeks there. I apparently met my neurologist Dr Swingler for half an hour and he said I was completely lucid during the meeting but I only realised I had actually met him when he told me about our meeting at my next appointment with him in Perth. I find it quite frightening that I have totally lost two weeks of my life but I'm comforted by the fact that my brain was allowed a two week holiday from the constant pain of my Dystonia and it was at a time when I really needed the break.

I arrived back in Moredun B in a taxi feeling much better and I apologised to the staff for my behaviour prior to my transfer even though I didn't know exactly what I was apologising for! I continued to progress and I was allowed out of the ward on several passes. I was on one such pass when I was filling in the details of who I wanted to be my nominated person. This is basically the person who, when I'm to unwell to do so, ensures that I'm being treated in accordance with the wishes expressed in my Advance Statement. The Advance Statement gives details of how I would like to be treated in the event of further manic episodes, including specific treatments I'm quite willing to have but also outlining treatments I specifically don't want. Anyway I had decided that I wanted my boss at work Olav to be my nominated person as he was also a good friend and I trust him implicitly. I didn't want my mum to do it because I thought it would make her 'piggy in the middle' between my Dad and I but I thought I better tell my Mum this so I phoned her to explain my reasons.

I thought she had understood why I was doing this but obviously not as when she had put the phone down she started crying. Dad came into the house, saw mum crying and put two and two together to get eight. Mum phoned me to say he had assumed it was me that had upset her and that he was already on his way down to the flat. I have to say I was a little scared at this prospect so I called my brother to tell him what was happening. When Dad arrived I was still on the phone to Scott and I made a point of not hanging up the call so he could listen to everything that was said.

There was a loud knock on the door and when I opened it I could see that Dad was fuming. He asked me what the hell I was playing at and despite my explanation about the nominated person he went through to the kitchen and got a knife with an eight inch blade. He stood right in front of me and lifted up his sweat-shirt saying "you may as well stab me through the heart now because you are ripping this family apart". I couldn't really believe that this is how he interpreted the recent events and my illness. He said that I better not hurt Mum again or I would have him to deal with. He also said that if I had enjoyed my time in Australia so much then maybe I should go and live there.

He continued on with his tirade about how he would do anything to protect Mum. It was only when he left that he realised that Scott had been listening to the whole conversation but he was only slightly perturbed by this. I on the other hand, because of my fragile mental state, was very shaken up by this confrontation so I got in my car and drove myself back up to Murray Royal. They were surprised to see me because I had been progressing so well but were very understanding when I explained what had happened. Now as far as I know my mother had never confirmed my accusations of psychological abuse to any of the staff at Murray Royal so that meant it was always just alleged abuse but when I told the nurse what had just happened I'm sure she realised that I had always been telling the truth even if I couldn't actually prove it.

At my pre- discharge meeting on the 16th of June 2008 I was anxious to ensure that what had happened with NHS 24 couldn't happen again and I was therefore keen to 'set in stone' an urgent referral pathway specific to me. I was basically told that I would have ample out-patient follow-up and therefore this would not be required. My short term detention order issued on admission had been revoked on 12th May 2008.

Unfortunately that evening I started to feel very anxious again so I decided to drive back up to Murray Royal. I rang the buzzer and two nurses came down to speak to me. Unfortunately I was told that as I had officially been discharged earlier in the day I would need to be referred by a doctor before I could get back on to the ward. The only way I could be referred as it was after hours was to phone NHS 24 again. You can imagine how distressing this was after what had just happened with my previous admission. Fortunately because I have such a good memory for numbers I could remember the NHS 24 number so I phoned it on my mobile. I explained what was happening to the lady who answered the phone but I don't think she could actually believe that I was standing at the front door of Murray Royal Hospital seeking assistance but nobody would let me in. Anyway I don't know if NHS 24 called the hospital but about fifteen minutes later the nurses came back down and I was allowed on to the ward for that night.

This was the last wobble I had after being discharged but because the service I had received from NHS 24 had been so poor I decided that I didn't want another mental health patient to go through what I had been through. Also despite the fact that I had been in the mental health system for sixteen years I did not know anything about Advance Statements, Community Psychiatric Nurses or Nominated Persons.

I phoned up the two main news channels in Scotland, the BBC and STV and managed to get them both to put my experience on the evening news as the lead story. Hopefully if this helped one person then it would have been worth it. It was not long before my latest manic episode had faded and I slumped back into my usual routine. It was probably too generous to even call it a routine as looking back it was definitely more of a rut.

CHAPTER SEVEN

Over the next few years my Dystonia was becoming more and more painful. Things that I had previously enjoyed became more and more of a struggle. Walking eighteen holes on the golf course became a form of torture and that was not just because the standard of my golf was slipping year on year. After every round I had to go and lie down for a couple of hours and I also hardly ever went up to the clubhouse for a drink with my playing partners now as I just wanted to go home and rest. Even driving to and from work was getting worse as my neck spasms pulled my neck to the right it was harder for me to drive safely.

As a result of all of the above I decided that I would now consider having the last course of treatment available to me. Unfortunately this treatment was also seen as a last resort as it involved brain surgery. I asked my neurologist to make a referral so I could at least take the first step and see the neurosurgeon based at Ninewells Hospital in Dundee. I also had to check that the placement of the electrodes in my brain wouldn't affect my Bipolar disorder. The psychiatrist confirmed that the surgery would not affect this so I went down to Dundee for my appointment with Professor Eljamel the surgeon. Ironically the first thing I had to do was undergo a psychiatric evaluation which I passed. I then saw professor Eljamel for no more than five minutes in which he decided that I would be a suitable patient for the surgery. Even though I had been given the green light and the pain I was having to endure daily was getting worse I chickened out and said to my Neurologist that I was going to wait a while until more operations had been carried out and therefore the surgeons would know exactly where to put the electrodes. My neurologist Dr Swingler thought that this was actually a sensible approach as the surgery was still really in its infancy.

I waited for a year and got to the point where I couldn't take the pain anymore. It was preventing me from playing golf and even driving too and from work had become an ordeal. Then towards the end of 2011 I was sitting in work when I took a ten pence piece out of my pocket and proceeded to toss it into the air at the same time asking my colleague Lisa to shout heads or tails. Lisa called heads and as I went to retrieve the coin I said to her that if it was heads I wouldn't have the brain surgery but if it was tails then I would. She off course didn't want to be responsible for such a major decision and quite rightly she said that I shouldn't be deciding it on the random toss of a coin. The coin landed on heads so I think I must have already made my mind up to have the surgery as that December, I told my neurologist to put me on the waiting list. I was told there was a waiting list of about six months. Now by the time six months had passed I had almost managed to put the surgery to the back of my mind so when I opened the letter telling me my operation would be in four weeks my stomach fell to the floor. I was now officially terrified.

The letter said that I was to phone and confirm that I could come into hospital on Friday the 6th of July for surgery on the Saturday. However when I phoned to confirm the professor's secretary told me that there had been a mistake on the letter and that I should come in on the 5th as I was due to get a scan on the Friday. She also said that the surgery was not on the Saturday but on the Monday. These administrative errors did not fill me with a great deal of confidence.

I realised that this operation was going to be very serious and that there was a chance that things could go wrong. I decided that I better get my affairs in order before I went under the knife as I had no idea if I would be capable of doing this after. I drew up an informal will which I gave to my Mum to be opened if I didn't survive the surgery. I made my Mum my Power of Attorney in case I was left unable to make decisions for myself. In this I also made it clear that if I was not able to look after myself independently then I was to be put in care as I didn't want my parents to have to spend the rest of their lives looking after me when they should have been enjoying retirement. I also signed an advance decision which stated that if during the operation my brain was damaged so much that I could not survive without artificial aids then I wasn't to be resuscitated. Before the operation I had also researched a place in Switzerland and an organisation called Dignitas because if I was left with no quality of life then I had arranged with my best friend Carl in Australia to come over and take me there to end my life.

It was, looking back, a blessing in disguise that I only had to wait four weeks for the operation as it didn't leave me with much time to dwell on it. My brother came up from Glasgow to see me before the operation and he asked me whether I was awake when the surgery took place. Now I had just assumed that it would be done under general anaesthetic but I was suddenly wondering whether I had got this wrong. I googled 'Deep Brain Stimulation' and the first item listed said that the patient was awake during surgery. The panic was now setting in as I knew I didn't have the bottle to do the operation without a general anaesthetic. I quickly sent an e-mail to Dr Swingler asking him to confirm that the operation was indeed carried out using a general anaesthetic. To my huge relief he confirmed that this was the case.

I rather optimistically decided to take three weeks off work to have the operation and recuperate. This was off course assuming that there would be no complications. I arrived at lunch time on the 5th of July at Ninewells with my Mum. I was admitted to ward 23B where I said hello to the patient in the bed next to me. He'd had brain surgery but they had nicked something on the way in which had left him temporarily blind in one eye. He was a very nice man as was the young man who was in the bed diagonally across from me. He had been rushed into hospital with fluid on the brain as far as I could gather but the operation to remove this had been a success even if he was still finding it difficult to find words when in conversation. The older gentleman across from me must have been expecting a five star hotel rather than an NHS hospital. I think his operation had been cancelled due to his fluctuating blood sugar levels so maybe that was why he wasn't in the best of spirits.

The next day I was not taken for my MRI scan until about 2.30pm and by the time I actually got to the high resolution MRI machine which was located in the bowels of the hospital it was probably after three. An intravenous line was put in my arm so that they could inject liquid in to me that would show up on the scan. The ladies at the machine were very nice but they realised very quickly that it was not going to be easy for me to keep my head still during the scan. They told me that usually patients having Deep Brain Stimulation (DBS) for torticollis have a general anaesthetic to keep their head still during the scan but I think professor Eljamel wanted to see if I could keep my head still enough without the need for an anaesthetic. I lay down at the throat of the MRI machine and my head was placed in a cage which had a mirror on the inside. I was given ear plugs to muffle the sound of the machine. I wish I had known that you could bring your own CD's with you to be played when you are in the machine. Then the ladies jammed my head into the cage with two blocks of polystyrene to try and keep my head as still as possible. Unfortunately if my head is jammed in place then my neck spasms against the objects holding it there. These spasms are even worse during stressful situations and this was certainly stressful. In my head I was thinking that if I don't keep my head still then there is a good chance that the electrodes will not be placed in the correct position in my brain. My head was now fighting against the polystyrene blocks and it was absolute agony. The ladies kept asking me if I was ok to continue and I kept saying yes as I knew I had to get through this procedure. I had an alarm button in my hand that I could have pressed at any time to stop the scan but I was now beginning to feel as if this was just another test from God that I had to go through if I was ever going to prove he existed. The only difference was that this time I was not having a manic episode. Finally the machine stopped shaking and the noise faded away and after about twenty five minutes I was pulled out. I knew before the ladies told me that I had not kept my head still enough but I was shocked to hear that I was now going to the other MRI machine upstairs to have another scan.

When I finally got to the machine upstairs it was twenty to five on a Friday afternoon and the nurse manning the machine gave me the distinct impression that he had somewhere he needed to be. He quickly jammed my head in the cage with even more polystyrene than before ignoring the fact that I was telling him that my head would fight against this saying that it was there to keep my head still. Unlike the previous scan he did not utter one word to me for the entire twenty five minutes that I was in the machine. In fact when the machine stopped I thought for one horrible moment that he may have gone home! Finally he withdrew me from the machine and opened the cage and to add insult to injury proceeded to sneeze over me. Before I left the room he told me that I would have to have the scan done again on Monday before my operation under general anaesthetic but I could have told him this anyway as I knew I had not been able to keep my head still.

This was the worst fifty minutes I had spent in my life and I can only advise other patients with Spasmodic Torticollis to insist that they have the scan done under general anaesthetic as I would hate them to have to go through what I did. I got back to the ward about five o'clock just as dinner was being served but as I was now gasping for a cigarette I nipped out for a couple of them as I was still feeling really shaky. I came back to the ward and had my fish and chips before phoning Mum to come and get me as I was given a weekend pass as there was no point in me spending Saturday and Sunday in the hospital. Mum picked me up and I was very glad to get back to my own flat even if it was only going to be for a couple of nights.

I returned to the ward on Sunday night around about six. Mum gave me a lift back to the hospital but as we were driving back I thought that she should know that the MRI scans had really shaken me up to the point where I was concerned about my mental state. I asked her to make sure that she kept a close eye on my mood over the next week as I didn't want to have to cope with the brain surgery and a manic episode at the same time. I had a new patient in the bed next to me when I arrived back on the ward but he was a very nice man who was getting the discs in his back operated on. There was also a young man across from him who was getting a similar operation. They had both been lorry drivers so I suppose a bad back was almost an occupational hazard. I have to confess that I didn't even realise that it was neurosurgeons that carried out back operations. I had assumed that they only operated on the brain. A young junior doctor came to speak to me about my operation and the risks involved before I signed the consent form. He told me that there was a 2% chance of a blood clot during surgery. At least I was first on the list for surgery the next day so I wouldn't have to hang about thinking of what might go wrong. I told the doctor that the last time I had major surgery I had needed a catheter on both occasions so he said that they would insert the catheter during surgery. I had assumed that the operation would take a few hours but I was told by the junior doctor that it wouldn't be that long. Obviously I would be under for longer because I now needed to have the MRI scan before surgery. The surgeons then took about forty five minutes to calculate exactly where the electrodes would go and then the operation itself would take another forty five minutes. It also took about the same amount of time to bring me out of the anaesthetic.

I didn't think I would get much sleep that Sunday night but too my pleasant surprise I slept well and woke up about seven o'clock. I took a shower and then got dressed in my 'bum oot' gown as I call it. I still haven't figured out why we all have to walk about with our backsides hanging out before surgery! I had been nil by mouth since nine the previous night but I wasn't really feeling like breakfast that morning anyway. I think it was about eight thirty when the theatre nurse came to wheel me to the operating theatre. For some reason there was a small voice in the back of my head that wanted to shout out stop as loud as I could but as in the MRI machine I felt that this was just another test and there was no going back now.

I was wheeled into the operating theatre holding area where a nurse went through a quick checklist with me regarding what I had eaten over the last twenty four hours and also any previous surgeries I had gone through. I was then wheeled into the main theatre where the anaesthetist wasted no time in putting me under. At least now everything was now out of my hands and I hadn't chickened out. My life was now in the hands of God and professor Eljamel.

Obviously I have no recollection of what happened during or after my surgery. I can only tell you that my Mum got a call telling her and Dad to get to the hospital as quickly as possible as there had been serious complications during surgery. After the electrodes had been placed in my brain I was put back into the CT scanner which showed a large dark area on the right side of my brain. I was rushed back into theatre where the surgeons worked to repair the clot. I have no recollection of coming round after surgery or being taken back to the ward.

When I did come round the next day my left side was completely paralysed and it was not just my arm and leg but also the left side of my face and throat. I had a lot of medication to take after the operation as I needed painkillers and drugs to prevent infection. Because of the weakness on the left side of my throat I was finding it very difficult to swallow so I had to take the numerous pills with yoghurts and iced water. The weight of the ice in the water helped to wash down the pills but I have to say that it was quiet sickly as one round of pills would require a whole yoghurt. I hadn't even had time to think about my twenty year, twenty five a day smoking habit as I was not well enough to go outside for a cigarette and the nurses were just putting nicotine patches on me anyway.

Mum and Dad said that the surgical team were devastated by the results of surgery but professor Eljamel had said that the electrodes were exactly where they wanted them to be. Professor Eljamel also told me during his rounds that he hoped my movement would start to come back as the swelling in my brain went down. However that afternoon during visiting time as I sat in front of my parents with drool coming down both sides of my mouth I apologised to them because they 'now had a vegetable for a son'.! We were all very emotional but they just gave me a big hug. I think that looking back that was definitely my lowest point because the next day as the swelling in my brain went down I started to get some movement back down my left side but this was where the hard work started.

CHAPTER EIGHT

There seemed to be quite a quick turnover of patients in the ward as now across from me was a nice guy who I think had been getting palliative care for cancer of the spine. What I do remember is that his wife and daughter were on their way to visit him one evening when an idiot dropped a hockey ball of the flyover over the Kingsway on to their front windscreen. Now his wife was going about fifty miles an hour but fortunately she resisted the temptation to slam on the breaks and hence managed to avoid a major pile up.

There was also a chap from Nairn who had epilepsy and he'd had deep brain stimulation to try and control this. When he had a fit his mum would wave a magnetic band over the machine in his chest which would immediately stop the fit. Unfortunately the machine in his chest had been malfunctioning so he was in to get it fixed. The fits he had were so serious and violent that he had put his head through solid wooden doors and even dented his dad's car while he was washing it and started fitting.

It was not long before I got my own set of wheels from Scott the Occupational Therapist. I got a comfortable wheel chair which was adjusted for my needs. My brother even managed to get me the proper gloves to protect my hands from the spokes. Unfortunately I had all the gear but I couldn't even drive it. As I still had no power in my left side I could only propel myself with my right hand which meant I only succeeded in going round in circles.

I also got in trouble with the nurses because I was trying to put my slippers on to go to the toilet when my foot slipped on the floor and I fell of my bed. Fortunately apart from a big bruise on my hip and also a bruised pride there was no damage done. I also managed to end up flat out on the bathroom floor one night too. I had been standing in front of the toilet bowl when my evening medication seemed to kick in all of a sudden and my legs went to jelly. I thought it was safer to just let myself slowly go to the floor rather than fight it and the nurses were by my side in seconds after I pulled the cord to attract their attention.

Now because of all the painkillers and other medications I was taking I had not had a bowel movement for days so I was given a couple of suppositories which were not pleasant at all as I felt like I had consumed a vat of vindaloo curry the night before. I was also left dangling over a bowl for what seemed like ages until basically the ring of fire was too much to bear and I asked to be lowered on to my bed again. I would advise others to prevent this from happening by taking slow working laxatives immediately after surgery and not to let it build up like I did and believe me the fact that it was brain surgery that I had just had didn't help as at times I felt as if the top of my head was going to pop off! Sorry about the graphic detail but in this case there is no such thing as too much information. Mind you I would also beware of when you start to feel the laxatives work as I was caught short on more than one occasion.

The next day Scott took me down to occupational therapy where he proceeded to give me a quick lesson on how to use my wheelchair. Immediately after my half an hour with Scott, Claire took me to physiotherapy where she put me through my paces getting me to sit and stand and stretch my muscles. Even though the movement in my left side was returning my brain had forgotten how to use my left side so I basically had to teach it all over again. Talking of teaching reminds me that while as I was in physiotherapy this lady was passing me using two walking sticks when she stopped and looked straight at me. She pointed one of her sticks at me and said

"Crawford Buchan". It was Mrs McKinness my primary one teacher who had recognised me after thirty seven years. I was curious to know what defining feature had jogged her memory and she told me it was my eyes.

After my physio David from occupational therapy took me next door so I could do some Biometrics. One of the other things the clot had damaged was my eye sight and I now had a very big blind spot on my left side. Now this blind spot was very disconcerting and dangerous as it did not present itself as a black area in my peripheral vision. It was just that my brain did not see things on the left hand side. I would have difficulty telling the time from a dialled clock face as my brain missed out the left hand side of the clock face so my Dad bought me a digital watch. If somebody left something on the left hand side of a corridor then I could walk straight in to it quite easily. The work with David was to try and improve this blind spot. I would sit at a computer screen and balls would fall from the top of the screen which I had to try and catch by moving a basket under them before they reached the floor. This game could also be used to improve the strength in my left hand as it was possible to increase the resistance on the handle I needed to turn to move the basket. The occupational therapy and physiotherapy were done in the afternoons on Monday to Friday but as there was none at the weekends it meant these seemed to drag on.

The therapies usually finished at about three in the afternoon just as visiting started so I was usually very tired when my parents arrived and therefore was not the best patient as I became irritable very quickly. Although I had now started to give up the cigarettes it was not long before I replaced it with another addiction. Mr Whippy ninety nine ice cream cones. There was a small shop in the hospital foyer that sold Mr Whippy ice cream and now every time Mum and Dad arrived I was desperate to be wheeled down to get my sugar fix. If it was a nice afternoon we would go outside and it was nice to finally feel the fresh air on my face. I also have to confess that despite having stopped smoking I liked the passive smoke I got in the area outside the front door. There was a message relayed every two minutes reminding people that it was a non-smoking area but this was ignored by most.

There was another smoking area that I had used when I first came into the hospital. I remember asking the nurse where the smoking area was and she showed me along one corridor before she said "just follow the bones". I thought she was being funny until I actually went along the corridor only to find painted on the wall were human bones which when followed led straight out past the porters to the patients smoking area. I felt guilty about smoking just before undergoing such major surgery so I limited the number of times I went out for a cigarette.

One of the not so nice results of the general anaesthetics and all the medication I was now taking was that the skin felt as if it had been removed from my tongue. I was unable to eat anything so my weight fell rapidly which wasn't really a bad thing as I could do with losing a few pounds. This could not go on for ever though so Mum started to bring me in some very soft bread sandwiches with a range of fillings from tuna with Worcester sauce to thinly sliced roast beef with coleslaw. I would eat these with some kettle crisps and too many cans of coke. When I say too many I mean that I was having trouble sleeping and I don't think the coke was helping.

At some point as the patients on the ward came and went the patient from hell moved in beside me. Now I had come into hospital prepared for snoring so I had bought a packet of ear plugs but you could not prepare for this man's snoring. Even with my music on at full volume and my ear plugs in I could not drown out the noise. He also kept leaving his zimmer at the side of his bed in my blind spot so I kept clipping it when I went to the toilet. Now I know that some people can't help the fact that they snore loudly but I soon realised that these consecutive nights of no sleep were taking a toll on me mentally. Because of my Dystonia I couldn't get comfortable in my bed and I don't think the nurses really understood the condition Spasmodic Torticollis as they kept saying "you don't look comfortable Crawford". I tried to tell them that comfortable was a word that had not been in my vocabulary for about twenty years.

The only thing that was actually keeping me sane at night was listening to music. Mum had bought me a small CD player but as I didn't actually own any CDs I asked her to buy me a double CD of Oasis's greatest hits as I knew I liked them. Unfortunately I had been using the CD player for about a week before I realised that you had to hit the off button twice to stop it so I had been going through batteries by the dozen. Eventually Mum started to buy me the ones where you could check manually whether they had any charge left in them and this probably cut my usage down by half.

As I was no longer smoking my sense of taste started to come back so unlike all the other patients I actually thought all the hospital meals were very good, especially the soups and the puddings. Amazingly I started to eat fruit which I had not really done before. I joked with my parents that professor Eljamel must have taken the oranges from the back of my brain and mixed them with the apples at the front and turned me into a fruit cocktail! I remember just how good that first Granny Smith apple tasted. It was a taste explosion on my tongue. I couldn't believe that I had chosen to deprive myself of these tastes for twenty years and not just that but wasted thousands of pounds at the same time. Mum brought me in a very juicy ripe peach and although most of the juice ended up on my t-shirt it tasted like nectar from the Gods.

One afternoon on the ward just before my parents left I was seen by Dr Gentleman who was the consultant at the Royal Victoria Hospital which specialised in brain injuries. He explained to me that the hospital was specifically used to treat patients with similar brain injuries to mine. There were only sixteen patients in the hospital so the treatment was much more intensive. Dr Gentleman explained that they were holding a bed for me in the unit until I had recovered from the second part of my surgery. The hope was that after I left the brain clinic I would be back to the same physical state as when I walked into NInewells to have my operation. This was all very positive even if it was going to take about four months in the hospital. I now couldn't wait to get off the ward and into my new home especially as my next door neighbour was not getting any better. I walked into the toilet one morning and it was obvious he had been smoking. At first I didn't know whether to report this or not but then I decided that it was not only me he could be endangering. I told Karen one of the nurses but asked her not to make out that it was me who had spilled the beans. She came and stood at the bottom of both our beds and basically gave us both a talking to about smoking in the toilets as she knew I was in the process of giving up so theoretically it could have been me. After she gave us both this verbal volley she turned to me and mouthed "I know it wasn't you".

I now just had to get through the second part of my surgery. This was where a small machine just bigger than a match box was placed in the left side of my chest and connected up to the electrodes in my brain using a wire which was routed under my skin and behind my left ear. When the machine in my chest was turned on it would send electric pulses to the electrodes and these were designed to stop the spasms in my neck at source. Although not as dangerous as the first operation this was still brain surgery as the surgeon had to open up the two holes he had already made in my skull to enable him to connect the wire to the electrodes. As I had now started to make a quick recovery from the first operation and the clot I was absolutely terrified at the prospect of this second operation now being even more aware of what could go wrong. As usual when faced with a difficult decision in my life I phoned my best friend in the whole world Carl. I had met Carl on my first trip to Australia and we had just hit it off from the first moment we met. If Carl had been a woman then I'm not ashamed to say that I would definitely have asked him to marry me by now. I phoned Carl on my mobile and he basically told me what I already knew on this occasion which was that I had come this far so I would probably always regret it if I didn't now go on and have the second part of the procedure. The man in the bed next to me was only interested in how much a forty minute phone call to Sydney on my mobile was costing me. I don't think he really knew what I meant when I told him it was priceless! When I was signing the first consent form I had made my mum promise that they would go ahead with the second part even if something terrible happened as I was terrified of being trapped in my own body unable to communicate my wishes. The thought of the surgeons deciding not to complete the procedure because the first part had gone wrong and therefore consigning me to a life of silent pain was one of my worst fears.

Before I officially agreed to have the second operation my Dad said that I had two choices. I could go to the brain rehab clinic right now and just decide not to have the second operation or I could have the second operation. I decided to ignore this option and take the attitude' in for a penny then in for a pound'. There was no going back now. The night before I had the second operation the same young doctor who had got me to sign the initial consent form came round. This time when he said there was a 2% chance of a blood clot I realised that this could happen to me again. Now some people would say that you would have to be very unlucky to get two clots from consecutive operations but as I said to my parents after the first one what makes me so special that I should expect to be part of the 98% that doesn't have a clot. I was still terrified though and that night I definitely said a big prayer. Mum also said that the local church in Gask had also said a prayer for me which was very nice. Unfortunately I was fourth on the list for my operation the next day so I was going to have to lie and think about it which I was not looking forward to.

I didn't get any sleep that night but that was down to the loud snoring beside me rather than worrying about the operation. It was half past eleven in the morning and I had been fasting since eight thirty the previous night when Mr considerate beside me asked if I had any kit-kat biscuits left. I reminded him rather sternly that I hadn't eaten anything for some time and he would be getting his lunch in half an hour anyway. The afternoon dragged on and on and I was still waiting to be taken to theatre. It was getting to the point where I thought that I may not get taken that day when at four o'clock the theatre porter came to get me. I think the nurses could see in my face how worried I was and a couple said good luck and they would see me again in a couple of hours.

It was the same theatre nurse Mitchel, I think his name was that went through the same checklist as my first operation. He obviously knew what had happened first time round and therefore he could understand the fact that I was terrified. He tried to reassure me that he would see me again on the other side of my anaesthetic. I was wheeled in and the same anaesthetist put me under. I have to say that to get put under was really great because I had not slept for the last few nights so this was actually what I needed as I was on the point of another manic episode if I had remained on the ward. Obviously I can't tell you anything about the operation other than to say it was a success and I was very emotional when I saw Mitchel on the other side and I was still in one piece. The entire theatre team were excellent and the anaesthetist even came to see how I was doing on the ward later that evening.

Professor Eljamel and Dr Gentleman had decided that it was sensible to wait until the machine in my chest had been switched on before transferring me to the Royal Victoria Hospital. This was to be done on Thursday. I think it was Tuesday that we got a welcome addition to the ward. Peter was admitted to the bed opposite me. He was in to have the discs in his back operated on. Now as soon as the man in the bed next to me heard this he said that was the operation he had come in for and now he couldn't walk! It takes quiet a lot for me to lose my temper these days but this was just too much along with the lack of sleep caused by you know who. I angrily pointed out that Peter didn't need to be told about this man's operation going wrong when he was facing something similar. I tried to reassure Peter by pointing out that the surgeon doing his operation was one of the best in the country and I had already seen patients getting similar operations have it one day and be out the next. It was refreshing to be able to have a decent conversation with a really nice guy for a change and I don't think it took Peter too long to realise why I was being driven up the wall by my next door neighbour.

I had tried to get myself moved after my second operation as I now realised how fragile my mental state was and so I told Karen the nurse that if I wasn't moved there was a very good chance I could have another manic episode. Karen unfortunately said that there was nowhere else to move me at the moment so when I came back from theatre I was horrified to find out I was going back in the same position as before. When I did return to the ward I should not have been amazed to find my next door neighbour offering me a cigarette! He was a forty a day man and had bought himself one of those battery operated cigarettes that light up when you inhale. He was at pains to point out that this had cost him thirty pounds as he said "now you just want a couple of draws don't you Crawford"? I declined the offer as I had just woken up from brain surgery.

I was now counting down the days until Friday as that is when I was to be transferred to the Brain clinic. On Thursday morning Kate the Dystonia Nurse Specialist came to see me to take me to get the machine in my chest switched on. I was very excited to see if this was going to transform my life and eradicate years of pain. In the room with Kate I was introduced to John who worked for the place in Minneapolis, The St.Jude Medical Centre, where the machine was made. He had come up on the train from Manchester to oversee the switching on off my machine and also the initial settings. I had no idea what to expect but I will try and explain it as best I can. A strap to transfer messages from the machine Kate had to the machine in my chest was placed over my shoulder so it covered the scar on my chest. Kate sat in front of me with a machine that looked like an ipad with a pen which she used to touch the screen of this ipad. John from time to time would lean over and say give him 1.5 volts there and then Kate would touch the screen with the pen. They would then both look at me intently which at first was quiet worrying as I didn't know if they were just waiting to see some visible sign of this electricity now going to the electrodes in my brain. Kate asked me to tell them if I felt the slightest sensation in my face no matter how small.

The first thing I felt was a slight tingling on the gum below my bottom teeth. Kate and John seemed encouraged by this and they added some more voltage. Suddenly my left hand formed a tight fist and no matter how hard I tried to open it I just couldn't. Although a bit scary these reactions were not at all painful and Kate was very reassuring when she said that they would take that clenched fist away.

Unfortunately it takes a bit of time for all the residual electricity in the brain to completely disappear so it was sometime before I could extend my fingers again. The idea behind the electric impulses now being sent to the brain was to try and give me dystonia in certain parts of my body so they could then take it away. For instance part of my Dystonia was the tremors I had in my left hand so they were giving this hand Dystonia so they could then take it away and therefore remove the tremor. They adjusted the volts again and I felt my left eyebrow start to droop but again this was taken away and it went back to normal. Then the whole of the right hand side of my face started to droop so I felt like Droopy the cartoon dog all of a sudden. Kate and John were now trying to move the Dystonia to the right side of my neck where the spasms were at their worst so they could then take it away and hence control the spasms. As they were doing this my lower jaw suddenly started to vibrate uncontrollably and after this reaction was removed Kate and John decided that this was probably enough for my first time. Unfortunately Kate pointed out that most patients, because of the severity of the operation, expected there to be a miracle cure when the machine was turned on for the first time but usually it took about six to twelve months of adjustments before the settings were where they needed to be to get the maximum benefits. Despite this I still felt better than I had done in the last twenty years. However I realised there was still residual electricity in my brain when I was eating my dinner later that evening. My left hand started to clench up again and this made it impossible to hold my fork correctly. I was not overly concerned about this as Kate had said that if anything like this happened I was just to get one of the nurses to contact her and she would make a further adjustment to the settings. By the time she came round the next day my spasms had settled down again so we decided to leave things as they were and if I had any problems at the brain clinic I was just to tell one of the nurses over there and she would come out and adjust the settings.

When I went to physio that afternoon the physiotherapists said they thought that I was standing straighter already but maybe I didn't notice it as much because my neck was still in spasm. As Claire was away on holiday Gordon ran me through my paces. Now Gordon was a small chap who was very nice but he was definitely old school when it came to physiotherapy which was the way I liked it. He had played football for Corby FC and as we were doing my exercises he asked me if I knew what the Chump effect was. I off course didn't even if I had felt like one on more than one occasion. He described it as that moment when a swimmer is in those last ten metres and he feels his main competitor on his shoulder. Does he fold or does he rise to the challenge. Thorpe the Australian swimmer certainly didn't suffer from this nor did Tiger Woods. Now the first Dystonic symptom I ever got was a slight tremor in my left hand so now that the machine had been turned on Gordon was determined to test this. He proceeded to get a jug of water with various sizes of cups and even some very small containers for measuring out medicine. He got me to fill these up to the top and pour the water from one cup into another and to do the same with the smaller containers. To my amazement even with Gordon's eagle eye watching my every move I managed this without hardly spilling a drop. He then got me to do a mini obstacle course throwing sandbags into a box before hoping over walking sticks placed about a yard apart on the floor and finally a quick slalom round some bollards. I did this fairly well apart from a pathetic effort with the sandbags which Gordon was quick to point out even if I think he had his tongue in his cheek when doing so. Yvonne and Liz were pleased with my progress and I was very grateful for their encouragement and help.

Now it is with some reluctance that I go back to my continuing bowel problems but hopefully this story will make you smile. As I was due to be transferred to the brain clinic in two days I thought it would be sensible to at least try and clear out my system before I went so I received another two suppositories from the nurse. Unfortunately they didn't work as quickly as before so I spent a couple of hours lying on my bed listening to my CD player. I was still in that position when Professor Eljamel and his team of doctors arrived on their afternoon rounds. They asked me how I was doing and I replied "I have had two suppositories stuck up my arse for the last two hours and I'm listening to a John Denver CD so what do you think"? Mum in her wisdom had brought me a John Denver CD which wasn't really my taste.

The good news though was that my next door neighbour was being discharged tomorrow and Peter and I couldn't wait. I couldn't take another morning watching Jeremy Kyle on TV as unsurprisingly he thought that this was top class entertainment. I just hoped that my mind could handle just one more night of no sleep as a manic episode was drawing ever nearer. There were now more signs of this as I was having strong religious beliefs again and the man in the bed next to me had become the devil himself. I was also having increased sexual arousal which was very uncomfortable when I had a catheter in! I was being aroused by some of the very attractive visitors to the ward. I was actually so worried about this last symptom I brought it to the attention of Ashley, one of the older nurses. She said I was turning a very small problem into a big one! I don't think she meant this literally but we still had a laugh anyway.

Somehow I managed to get through that night but when I got up the man in the bed next to me was shouting at the nurses complaining that he was in absolute agony. I suddenly had an awful thought that he may not be well enough to be discharged. However when his son arrived after lunch to pick him up he made a miraculous recovery and jumped out of bed. In the morning to my astonishment he offered to come and visit me in the brain clinic but I politely said that wouldn't be necessary as I didn't expect to be there too long.

As his son wheeled him out of the ward door I raised my hands in celebration. Mum told me off for this but she really had no idea what that man had put me through since his admission. His bed wasn't empty for long and was filled by a very nice man called Luke. The whole atmosphere in the ward had changed as now we had Peter, Luke and Paul. I'm not entirely sure what was wrong with Paul but it was obviously very serious as he couldn't get out of bed or communicate verbally. I did ask him one day if he wanted a piece of my Cadbury's caramel bar and he nodded so I gave him a couple of pieces. It was immediately after this that I realised I shouldn't have done this as I didn't know what his allergies were or even if he was allowed chocolate. I confessed all to one of the nurses but she just told me not to do it again but there was no harm done on this occasion.

I quickly discovered from Luke that he was a keen pigeon racer a hobby that had always fascinated me as I had always wondered how the pigeons knew how to get home. Luke explained that it was basically a sixth sense although sometimes this went a little awry as he had recently been over to France for a race but only four out of eight of his pigeons returned. I asked him if there was much money to be made in the hobby and he said that some of the prize money was pretty good but that was obviously not what attracted him. I also asked him if he had a favourite pigeon and he said he did. It was called 'Frankie's Boy' and was named after a close friend of his that had died and you could tell that it really meant a lot to him. Unbeknown to me there was a Grand National for pigeons and 'Frankie's Boy' had come fifth winning Luke five hundred pounds in prize money but it was the place that mattered more. Luke also explained that there was usually quiet a lot of gambling on the races but he usually only put fifty pence on. That afternoon I found a fifty pence piece on the floor of the ward next to my bed. I was sure it wasn't mine so I said to one of the nurses that someone else must have dropped it. They decided it wasn't theirs so I gave it to Luke and asked him to put it on 'Frankie's Boy' in next year's Grand National and if we won any money then we would split it and donate it to a charity of our choice.

Finally I had a night to look forward to where there was not going to be the sound of ten growling bears five feet from my ear. Even though the ward was now quiet I think his departure had come too late to save my mental state as I still couldn't get to sleep that night but at least I had my transfer to the Royal Victoria to look forward to. I knew now that my mental state was beyond normal medical intervention because I was starting to have very strong religious beliefs again. When this happened I felt that if given the chance then I could prove that God existed. Unfortunately I thought that God had let everyone else I met in on this master plan and therefore they all knew I could prove this world changing discovery.

That morning I went to get the papers for Luke and Peter as it was good practice for my blind spot to be able to go down to the shop in the hospital foyer get these and come back with the right amount of change. The previous day I had also gone but it only confirmed how bad the blind spot was as I walked straight past the main paper stand at the front of the shop just because I hadn't even seen it. When I asked the girl at the counter where the papers were she looked at me as if I was some sort of alien as she couldn't believe I had walked straight past them. The fact that I did manage to get back to the ward safely with the correct change did improve my confidence though.

I was to be transferred to the brain clinic shortly after lunch and the nurse told me that all my paper work had been completed for my transfer. As my transfer time got closer I was getting more and more paranoid and I now confided in Peter that I was convinced that I wasn't actually being transferred to the brain clinic but they were going to take me to Carse View the mental hospital close by. Because of my past experience with this place I was terrified at the thought of this. Peter suggested we go down to the foyer for a Mr Whippy ice cream and as I wanted to occupy the time until the porter came to take me to the ambulance for transfer I jumped at this suggestion. As I also trusted Peter and thought he was obviously one of God's good guys trying to help me I had no reason to think this wasn't a good idea. I think Peter also realised my mind was going as he couldn't really understand why I thought I was going to Carse View when the nurse had just said I was getting transferred to the Victoria. I asked for a medium cone without a flake as I was still stuffed after lunch but the lady gave me a large cone with a flake. This was the second time she had done this and at first I thought it was because she felt sorry for me but then I realised it was just because she was a very nice person.

The trip for the ice creams had taken my mind of things for a few minutes but I still thought that everyone else knew that I was the person God had put on this Earth not only to prove he existed but also by doing so to clean up today's society which was totally out of control. God did not create Man and this beautiful Earth for us to behave as badly as we currently do. So when the porter came up to get me I thought the reason he was so nice to me was because he was also part of the bigger plan. I said my goodbyes to Peter, Luke and all the nurses thanking them for looking after me so well. The only problem with the porter was that he was a Dundee fan. Despite this I suggested that maybe one day we could meet up in Perth before the football for a bar lunch in the Cherrybank Pub.

After a short wait my designated ambulance driver was ready to take me on the short drive up to the Royal Victoria. Even at this late stage I was still terrified that the driver may just take me straight to Carse View. The drivers name was Scott, I think, and he also was very nice. I would later find out that Jane one of the nurses at the brain clinic was a relative of his. We had a nice chat on the journey up to the clinic and before I knew it to my relief we arrived at the Royal Victoria. It was a fairly old building which actually looked out over the cemetery but I didn't look upon this as a bad omen. I was just so glad to finally be there.

CHAPTER NINE

The first nurse to welcome me to the Hospital as I stepped of the ambulance was Scott's relative Jane. She was very nice and immediately made me feel very welcome and at ease. I was then shown to my room which was right at the end of the main corridor on the right. I was on a ward if you could call it that with three other patients Ali, Colin and Chris. My space was first on the right. It was great as it was my own private area with ample storage space and privacy if I wanted it, by pulling the curtain across the front. The nurse said that the Doctor would be along to chat to me shortly and immediately my stomach started to churn as I was still convinced that when they found out about my mental state I would be transferred to the psychiatric hospital. In the mean time I put up all the get well cards I had transferred from the hospital with me and they made my living space feel a bit more personal.

After the nurse had booked me in the doctor came in to see me. Her name was Emma and she was very nice. Before I had always tried to hide what I was feeling from the doctors for fear of being sectioned but this time despite the very real fear of going to Carse View I decided that I would just tell Emma the truth. Now I know if you have never suffered from a mental illness it is very difficult to imagine but I was now already having a manic episode. Now you may think why didn't I just tell the doctor that. Unfortunately when I start to feel an episode coming on my mind tries to fight as hard as possible to keep me from being in the best place for me which is obviously a psychiatric ward. I know that is crazy but that is the truth.

Believe me it would be a lot easier if I could just say take me to Murray Royal now and get my treatment started.

The other thing I should point out is that because of my manic episode I was now paranoid and I saw everyone as either good or evil and this was like black and white with no chance of any grey. After telling Emma about my beliefs and the fear that I was going to be transferred to Carse View I quickly formed the view that she was definitely good. She quickly reassured me that they had no intention of sending me to Carse View and she felt that my mental state was very good even if I did need to catch up on some sleep. I was very emotional as I felt that for the first time a doctor was actually listening to what I had to say about God and not just assuming it was my mental illness rearing its ugly head again. This may have been because Emma had just finished a placement on a psychiatric ward and in her opinion there was no need to send me to one!

I hadn't met anyone on the ward yet as they all had their blue curtains pulled across their bed spaces but as I was coming back from the toilet I met Ali, who was in the bay next to me, his daughter and wife. I introduced myself and they were all very nice. Ali I found out later was from Libya but he had been hit by a bus in Dundee and that is why he was on the ward. A nicer man you would be hard pushed to find. After navigating the first hurdle which in my head was Emma I made my way to the TV room. The tables were all set out for dinner. I took a seat at the end of the table directly across from Ali. The food was giving of an extremely appealing smell. Ali was having a pasta Bolognese so I asked him if he would recommend it. When he nodded I asked the nurse if I could have the same as it was table service in this hospital would you believe. I don't think I had realised just how hungry I was until I took the first bite. The pasta was delicious so I thanked Ali for his recommendation.

The dining area was now full of the other patients and it was quite nice that we all ate together like one big family. I can't really remember what I had for dessert but the food was much better than Ninewells and I was beginning to think that compared to ward 23B this was like a five star hotel although the standard of nursing was very high in both hospitals so far. The main thing was going to be whether I could get a good night's sleep in my new surroundings.

I went to bed that night more in hope than expectation as I knew that when in a manic state even if I hadn't slept for six straight nights combined with brain surgery my mind refused to switch off. That first night I did get about three hours sleep which I knew was never going to be enough to reverse my slide into a manic phase. Unfortunately for me Ali had a talking clock which kindly reminded me every hour throughout the night what time it was and also just how slow time was ticking by. When I did wake up I did feel refreshed and grateful for the three hours of shut eye as this was the first time my brain had got a rest since I had been anaesthetised for the second operation. However it was a catch twenty two situation as now my mind had rested it was again working overtime and looking for its next project.

It was not long before it found it. In my personal area there was a space with a desk and chair. On the desk was a dark red diary which had 201269 in big digits on a sticker on the front. Of course in my mind everyone now knew that for some reason God had chosen me to prove he existed so the first thing that came in to my mind when I saw the diary was. How did they know I was coming! Now looking back this is quite funny as I now of course realise that all new admissions got a diary with their date of birth on it. The trouble was I now thought that this was some sort of test and I assumed that I had to do my best to fill in the whole diary.

I sat down at the table and began to fill in all the usual details like address, phone number, place of work etc. Because I have a semi photographic memory I even started to fill in the phone number and fax number of a couple of Broxwood's main customers. I then tried to fill in the birth dates of all the family members I could remember but I have to confess I struggled with those of my sister's three girls and also my brother's daughter.

My memory is slightly sketchy over what I filled in next but I think it was the dates of the St Johnstone games that had already taken place since my hospital admission with the final scores, goal scorers and times plus a guesstimate at the possible crowd. I realised that I had stuffed this up with regard to the dates so I had to start again in the correct part of the diary. After this I decided to fill in the diary days from the date of my admission on the 5th of July to the day I was transferred to the brain clinic. Now to try and remember what I had for breakfast, lunch and dinner each day was very difficult if not impossible and also there was only limited space under each date to put in all the information. I suddenly had a Eureka moment to tackle the lack of space. I would use txt letter abbreviations to describe certain things that I had on a regular basis. For instance CB was not Crawford Buchan but Cornflakes and Banana. WRWJ was 'white roll with jam'. I also chuckled at this as obviously BC stands for before Christ and maybe it could now stand for before Crawford but there was an awful long road to walk before that ever happened and I could see that a lot of people would think this was very arrogant of me but if I didn't believe it how could I expect anyone else too. I had abbreviated a mug of white coffee with sugar to MWCWS but as I always had this I was very pleased with myself when I came up with the idea to just write MU standing for My Usual.

Obviously this diary in the hands of anyone else would be complete rubbish unless they were maybe a world war two code breaker. Even so in my head the diary was now very important as it was telling my life story from entering Ninewells to where I was now. It would also mean that I could write down what had and was happening and hopefully free up some much needed brain space as it was definitely overloaded at the moment. I'm not sure of exactly when I met the respective doctors but I do know that the next one I met was called Graeme and he was an extremely nice man. I got the feeling that despite the psychiatric experience Dr Emma had Dr Graeme really understood what I was going through even if this did not stretch far enough to believing that I could prove God existed!

Colin and Chris were housed at the far end of my ward where there was the toilet/shower room and a flat screen TV. I think it was the Sunday night and they were watching Hannibal on the TV. You don't really want to hear about people getting part of their brain cut off and fried and eaten when you are barely hanging on to sanity yourself. My brain had already been fried although not literally as the film depicted. I was going to bed but I could clearly hear the television and one of the characters was called Crawford which was really making my mind work overtime. I asked them to turn it down a bit and they kindly obliged but to be perfectly honest it was not going to make much of a difference to my sleep pattern.

I felt bad about asking them to turn the TV down so I took them up some ginger nuts. Now one of my relations believes that not only are ginger nuts the best dunking biscuit ever invented but also that they are a cure for any ailment. This only applies if they have been purchased from Marks & Spencer's. She did like the finer things in life which is not a bad thing if you can afford them. Mum on the other hand bought a cheaper brand of ginger nut which was still good but just not as good.

I still had some of each kind left over so I decided to do the ginger nut test on them both where I wanted them to tell me which brand they preferred. It was only after that I realised how stupid I had been because if either of them had a nut allergy then I could have killed them. If both of them had died I could have become the first ginger nut serial killer! For anyone who is still interested in the results of the test then Chris didn't give me a response but Colin definitely preferred the Marks & Spencer ones. He obviously had good taste because so do I.

As I was going to say before, despite the noise from the television being reduced I didn't really get anywhere near enough sleep. At least the weekend was now over as this could certainly drag as there was no Occupational or Physical therapy to break up the day. On Monday afternoon I had occupational therapy from Sophie who was a really nice lady. I was asked to make some toast and a cup of coffee. It may not seem that big a deal but all these things had to be done to ensure it was safe for me to be allowed home. I managed the toast and coffee without any problems and as a result Sophie suggested that I come down and make a bacon butty next time which sounded like a therapy I would be more than happy to participate in. I asked her if she was a red or brown sauce girl!? I explained that I sometimes had two bacon rolls at the weekend so I could then have one of each. I started to tell her that most weekends I would also grill an Asda breakfast pack with a tomato and fried egg. Sophie pointed out that she did not think the NHS would stretch to this! Before we finished I had another go on the biometrics video game that I had first tried with David in Ninewells. Sophie turned up the resistance on the handle used to move the basket at the bottom of the screen and got me to use my weak left hand to ensure this was getting a work out. I was still missing a few balls falling from the left of the screen but I had definitely improved since I first tried this exercise.

After my half hour with Sophie it was straight on to physiotherapy with Claire. I explained that one of my main goals after recovery was to be able to play golf again. Because of this she started me off on the balance pad. On the physio bed in front of me was placed an electronic set of scales. Standing from a sitting position I had to try and get my weight spread evenly over both feet. I could tell if I had succeeded if the green light on the electronic scale lit up. There were seventeen lights in total and the green light was the ninth light. Straight away I was able to get the light within one of the middle and I think Claire was quite impressed by this. Because of the weakness I still had in my left side she wanted me to make sure that most of my weight was on this leg when standing and by doing this the green light started to light up more often than not when I stood up. Because the golf swing finishes with most of the weight on the left leg Claire wanted to know how far over I could get balancing on my left leg. I was a bit sheepish at first but I then built up my confidence and was able to get all the way over to the third light from the left hand side of the scale. The session really felt like a golf lesson to me and I was thrilled that I could transfer my weight so easily during my first session.

I was now however shattered after no sleep for so many days and these two back to back sessions. Claire got me to spread out on the physio bed to do some stretches but I had to tell her that there was a good chance I may fall asleep due to my recent insomnia. I think she may have thought I was joking but this was only because she was not fully aware of my recent sleep deprivation. I was very happy that the physio was going to be concentrated on things I wanted to get back to and that the exercises would be adjusted to incorporate my golf. I knew that the brain clinic was the best place to treat my brain injury but unfortunately it wasn't the best place to treat my sleep deprivation.

When I went back to the day room I was now absolutely shattered. My brother and his wife and eldest son James were due to be visiting me in about ten minutes. They had been up North on holiday and were stopping of on their way back down to Glasgow. My primary school teacher was in the dining room. I was talking to her while texting on my phone and not really looking where I was going. Suddenly my left trainer caught on the radiator on the wall. Because I was so exhausted I had lost concentration which had me now tipping forward. As I fell I grabbed the back of a chair but only succeeded in pulling it with me. I could now see the hard wooden floor speeding towards my forehead. At the last moment I managed to turn my body and my shoulder caught the brunt of the impact with my head only getting a small bump. As I started to fall my primary school teacher started to scream for some assistance so fortunately the nurses and a doctor were there in seconds. Claire the physio had also been passing the door and heard the commotion so she was by my side as well. I can't tell you the doctor that examined me as I was pretty shaken up and my only concern was whether I had done any more damage to my brain. The doctor made me follow their finger with my eyes and came to the conclusion that I had escaped unharmed. I was still shaking like a leaf and that was when I saw my brother and his family walking to the front door.

They immediately saw how shaken I was but I now felt angry with myself because I had been looking forward to their visit so much and because of this stupid fall I had now ruined it. The nurse suggested I go and have a lie down as my legs were still like jelly. Scott, Sue, James and I walked back up to my personal space and I lay down on the bed. Sue was sitting on the seat closest to me with Scott and James at the foot of the bed. Sue is an absolute diamond and she could sense how upset I was. She asked me if I wanted a cuddle but I said if she did that I would start crying. She of course said that this was perfectly normal but I informed her that if I started I wouldn't stop. She again said that this would be fine but I didn't want to cry in front of James even if he was mature enough to show genuine empathy for my condition. The emotion did get the better of me though and I did have a wee cry but all I could think of was that song "Cry me a River" as that is what I think I really needed to do. I now had images of me at one end of the bed and this Tsunami coming out of my eyes!

Scott and family did not stay that long as they sensed I was upset and just wanted to be left alone to deal with my demons. I think it was at this point that one of the nurses came up to comfort me and the second she put her arm around me all the emotions I had been bottling up came flooding out. As this was really the first time I had properly cried since my initial symptoms of Dystonia twenty years ago it was, as you can imagine, a tremendous relief but now that the damns defences had been breached it was going to be difficult to stop the flow of emotions from becoming a raging torrent.

Now my mental state hadn't improved any during the day and I was still no nearer to being able to sleep. Now the name of this book as you know is 'Footprints in the Sand'. This comes from a small card that was in the back of the tiny small New Testament Bible that had fallen open to Matthew chapter 25 all those years ago in 1998. The card had the following message on it which comes from Isaiah 41:13 which reads as follows:-

One night a man had a dream. He dreamed he was walking along the beach with the Lord. Across the sky flashed scenes from his life. For each scene, he noticed two sets of footprints in the sand; one belonging to him, and the other to the LORD.

When the last scene of his life flashed before him, he looked back at the footprints in the sand. He noticed that many times along the path of his life there was only one set of footprints. He also noticed that it happened at the very lowest and saddest times of his life. This really bothered him and he questioned the LORD about it "LORD, you said that once I decided to follow you, you'd walk with me all the way. But

I have noticed that during the most troublesome times in my life, there is only one set of footprints. I don't understand why, when I needed you most, you would leave me."

The LORD replied "My precious, precious child, I love you and I would never leave you. During your times of trial and suffering, when you see only one set of footprints, it was then that I carried you"

Now I could associate this card closely with my own life especially since my first hospital admission in 1998. The scariest part for me was always when there was only one set of footprints behind me because I believe that the gift I have been given is to prove that God exists. Now I have been told throughout my journey that it is impossible to do this and when I have been asked how I'm going to do it I can only respond by saying that I'm willing to sacrifice myself to prove that God exists. Now this is truly terrifying because I did not want to die then or now but how can I possibly do anything to stop this happening if the Holy Father decides that my time on this Earth is up. Also I don't want to face my judgement day having failed to use the talent given to me and therefore be cast out into the darkness. Now as like the rest of this book you can decide whether I'm telling the truth or not and then you have to decide what does this mean if it is true. Well I just think it simply means that 'God walks among us' and I'm his vessel to teach society how to behave again. I think that basically God who created this Earth and all the beautiful creatures on it has had enough of watching all his hard work being ruined by War, famine, rape, murder and a society who believes that there will be no consequences for their actions.

In a society where prison is no longer a deterrent and even the death penalty does not stop abhorrent crimes from taking place. I personally think the only way we can change societies ways is for humans to realise that there is a heaven and their own actions during life will decide whether they go there on Judgement Day.

Until recently I also believed in hell but now I just believe that rather than going to hell death will just mean the end and we will not attain eternal life. The thought of spending all of eternity in the darkness would certainly make me think twice about doing something stupid again especially since the alternative is such an appealing one. Now obviously I can't tell you what Heaven is like but I think I can almost certainly say that it will surpass even our wildest dreams.

Now you like me at this point will be asking why God chose 'Crawford Buchan' out of all the tremendous men and woman that have graced the planet before him. I can't answer that question as I ask myself that every day. Believe me I'm no more special than the next man and excuse my French but my shit does not smell any sweeter than the next man either as I will prove to you later in this chapter. I have made numerous mistakes in my life and continue to do so daily but I like to think that I learn from them. Only God can perform miracles so do not ask me to make the crippled walk. I can only offer comfort and empathy without pity. I will try to be the best person I can be each and every day and if I can do that then I will sleep easy at night. My friends and family are still the most important thing in my life but if I'm not busy and a friend needs me then if I can be there I will be. I'm loyal and like my friends to be likewise. I do not hold grudges as life really is too short and forgiveness can cleanse the soul and heal open wounds. I'm never going to be perfect so mistakes are inevitable. I will try not to hurt those close to me and I will also not make promises I can't keep. If you ask me a question I will answer it to the best of my abilities and with the God's honest truth as I certainly believe that the truth will set you free.

My mental state in the brain clinic was now even more fragile to the point where I was terrified when visiting time was over and I knew I would have to face the rest of the night on my own. The lack of sleep and continual mental torture made me feel as if I couldn't take any more of this. As the pills prescribed by Dr Emma were not getting me off to sleep I was becoming more and more agitated. The exact sequence of events at this stage is somewhat blurred but rest assured that the events themselves did actually happen. I could not see me getting any respite from my over active mind unless I took some drastic action. I decided that I would get a taxi and get it to take me to Carse View the ICPU in Dundee where at least they would inject me with enough medication to knock me out. The brain clinic was not prepared to do this because I had just had brain surgery and a high dose of sedative medication could hide underlying problems from this. I was next seen by one of the doctors from Carse View Hospital in Dundee. I had spent three weeks in this unit in 2008 but I have to say I have no recollection of this as I was on so much medication I was not conscious of anything that was going on around me. Despite this I had met my Neurologist in the unit for half an hour and carried out a completely lucid conversation! I had absolutely no recollection of this meeting until my next appointment when Dr Swingler reminded me off it. The psychiatrist who came to see me in the brain clinic next was an Indian doctor and I tried to give her a rundown of everything that had been happening. I told her that I had been terrified that because I had tried to commit suicide this would automatically mean that I would go to hell when I died. It may have been as a result of her Indian background but she said that in some religions suicide did mean a fast track to the fires of hell. Needless to say this did not help to put my mind at rest!

My mood was also dependent on which nurses were on duty at night as like any workforce some were better at their jobs than others. My favourites were Jane, Lynn and Shirley or Denise and I referred to them as the dream team. If they were on duty I knew I could get through the night. In fact on one occasion I had decided that I was going to go home with Mum and Dad rather than stay another night but Jane had persuaded me to stay as she promised me that they would watch over me all night. Now the bad nights were when Elspeth and another male nurse were on duty as the male nurse was basically cruel even if he couldn't stop himself doing it. Elspeth who called all the patients cuddles as I think she could sense that we all needed a big cuddle was fantastic. She also knew how scared I got during the night and she promised to watch over me until the morning which meant an awful lot to me.

One day she was helping me get dried after my shower but after she had dried my feet she moved her head upwards just as I moved down so our heads collided. You could hardly call it a collision as our heads barely touched but within seconds there was a lump appearing on my head. This gave me a big fright as it showed how fragile my skull still was. I felt worse for Elspeth though as she was more upset than me but I tried to tell her that it was just an accident and these things happen. As for the male nurse well in my mind he had become my main tormentor. Fortunately I have a very strong mind so I knew what he was doing. On one occasion when I was having spasms on the right hand side of my body caused by residual electricity from the electrodes he came to my bedside and said "Crawford the machine in your chest isn't even switched on". Now you can imagine my reaction to this as I suddenly thought the staff in this clinic don't even know what operation I have had.

Now I have also always had a bashful bladder since I was a boy and can't pass urine at the urinals or sometimes even if I'm in a locked cubicle. Now this nurse knew this because when I told him I was in pain because I couldn't pass urine and wanted to have the catheter that had been removed after my surgery put back in he said that there would not be anybody to carry out this procedure for another three hours. Now if you have not had a catheter put in then you can't comprehend the pain that mounts up as the bladder fills up so three hours feels like a lifetime of pain. The nurse also said he needed a urine sample to check for infection but instead of giving me one cardboard container to fill up he gave me two cardboard containers to fill up. I remember joking with him that only God could fill up two containers! I only managed one and three quarters but for a little joke I filled the second one right to the top with tap water. The nurse was very surprised to see both containers full but as I always tell the truth I admitted to my ruse and of course both samples were poured down the sink as they were now useless. Now I can't prove it but I was also convinced that he was moving my mobile phone to cause me even more mental distress. I was leaving my phone behind my computer so I would know if it had been moved but when I came back to my bed it had been moved to my desk. I looked the nurse square in the eyes and asked him if he had been moving my phone and reminded him that he was answering in the eyes of the Lord. He of course denied it and Elspeth backed him up saying he was not like that. Elspeth didn't know that earlier that evening I had got my Dad to put the fear of death into him if he didn't stay away from me during the night so he certainly had motive as apart from God who was going to know what he had done.

I was having another panic attack where my strong religious beliefs were starting to terrify me. I went outside the clinic to make a phone call. Now I don't know if you have ever had a moment in your life where you have one chance to phone a friend but you have to select that friend from the list of contacts carried in your mobile phone. Well this is how I felt sitting outside the clinic but as I was looking for some inspiration a taxi pulled up outside. On the side of the taxi there was a website address www.biggart-baillie.co.uk which just happens to be the address of the law firm where my brother works in Glasgow. So not surprisingly I dialled Scott's home number but when his wife answered the phone the answering machine started making a horrible whistling noise. Despite Sue telling me that this would go off in a minute or two I was terrified that I was going to get cut off. Eventually the whistling stopped and I had a long conversation with Sue. By now my mental state was deteriorating so fast that I didn't know who to trust so when Sue suggested I tell the nurses I needed to see a doctor I began to question even her loyalty. Sue basically left me no choice as she made it clear that if I didn't speak to a nurse she would. Even though I was still very scared I asked to see the doctor.

Later in the evening when I was at my lowest ebb I said to Dr Gentleman that I felt like running down the corridor and diving head first of the hospital steps onto the tarmac below. He off course advised me this was not a very good idea but he was a bit flippant as he didn't seem to realise that I was deadly serious. In the meantime he handed me a long thin box. On the outside of the box was a letter from my sister saying she was thinking of me and had made another batch of her homemade cookies. Now Shuna's home made chocolate chip cookies are the best cookies in the world. I know I'm biased because she is my sister but I think if she gave the recipe to Marks & Spencer they would sell tons of them and she even wraps them professionally with a wee tie at the top. I gave most of the cookies away to various people including, Stevie and Katrina who were visiting Bruce who occupied the bed across from me. I had taken to Bruce from the first moment I met him. I was telling him about my travels to Australia when he told me he had cycled there. I laughed thinking he was pulling my leg but he was serious. You could see his brain straining to remember the route he took and slowly he began to remember country after country. Bruce at some point in his life had ended up in Laos where he had met his soul mate and wife Amphony who had given him two beautiful children.

Whenever his children visited Bruce's face lit up immediately and you could see his family were his world. I at this point dreaded every time my Mum and Dad left me at the end of visiting time as I knew that I had to battle against all the demons inside and outside my head on my own with only my faith to keep me going. Mum had been gently stroking my back in an attempt to calm me down enough to sleep but it was now too late as only a high dose of medication could do that. The gentle rub of my Mum's hand on my bear back stopped and when I turned around to face the ward entrance my Mum and Dad had gone. I was on my own again.

Now because I was terrified that I was going to have a similar episode as that suffered in the American psychiatric ward where I felt as if my body was re-enacting my car crash I had got the nurses to put padding on the wall next to my bed. I was terrified that if I had such a fit again that I would bang my head of the wall. For some reason I could not stop thinking about the young lad in the ward in Ninewells who had also had Deep Brain Stimulation to cut off the extreme epileptic fits he suffered. Now these fits were so bad he could put his head through a solid wooden door and he had done so on three occasions. I got it into my head that I was going to have one of these fits and bang my head of the wooden partition that separated our living areas. Obviously this would not be a good idea at the best of times but just after brain surgery the thought was enough to terrify me. On a couple of occasions the nurses had to physically stop me banging my head of the partition.

In my head I was convinced that I was the one God had chosen to change the world we live in and the nurses who were nice to me knew this. The nurses who were not nice to me thought because of what I had been chosen to do that I somehow thought I was special. In my head God now wanted me to show them that I wasn't any better than anyone else. This was another test and these tests always made me feel very anxious not knowing what I would have to do and also whether I would have the courage to carry them out. I went to the toilet which was in the corridor between the ward and the television room. When I got in there I took down my trousers to have a number two but as I was about to sit down on the toilet seat I couldn't help but see that the last person had left a massive turd floating in the toilet. Now obviously I didn't want to do this because it was repulsive but I had to prove that my shit did not smell any sweeter than the next man! I bent down and grabbed the turd with my right hand and proceeded to smear it all over my backside. I felt like throwing up but as the purpose of the test was to prove a point I instead pulled the cord to get the nurses attention. Three nurses quickly knocked on the toilet door so I let them in and showed them my hand covered in shit. They asked what had happened so I told them that I had done it to clear the toilet bowl. They off course told me that this was not my job and in future I should just leave it. After they had helped me to clean myself up and were leaving I said "my shit does not smell any better than the next man". I think one of them chuckled but I don't think they really understood what I was trying to tell them.

This was the most repulsive of the tests that I felt I had to carry out on the ward. One of the more amusing involved the cardboard boxes that were used to collect urine samples. I finally got my catheter removed when I had been so desperate to pee that I had actually urinated over the sides of the tube on to my pyjama bottoms. It was such a relief to get the tube removed but after removal you usually have to give a sample of urine to prove that you are capable of passing urine without the catheter. Now because of my mental state one of the symptoms of a manic episode is increased sexual arousal and I was certainly feeling this. So much so that it felt as if I had not had sex in years which actually was the truth. Anyway rather than give the urine sample required I somehow convinced myself that a semen sample was required! After such a long time, combined with my now intense sexual feelings it was not long before I was able to give a semen sample. The most amusing bit though was the nurse's face when I told her that I had produced a semen sample rather than a urine sample! Priceless. Off course I then was still required to produce the urine sample so I can tell you that the nurse that I handed that to was very glad that it was a urine sample this time!

By the end of the first week in the clinic I was starting to deteriorate very fast and I began to avoid situations that made me feel vulnerable or uncomfortable. For instance just before my occupational therapy I saw a police man entering the nurse's station. I suddenly thought that God might test me by getting me to kill someone for him and then I would have to spend the rest of my life in prison. The fact that there would be many knives at occupational therapy also added to my anxiety. Now obviously the thought of this terrified me but as I also knew I could not refuse the tests God put in front of me I decided not to go to the class. I could only control certain things and whether I went to the class or not was one of them so I decided not to go. For similar reasons I also decided not to go to my physio class either.

I had really lost track of the dates by the time my lack of sleep finally took over me but I think that I had only been in the brain clinic for a week so it may well have been Friday morning when I was finally tipped over the edge. I was lying on my bed when I became convinced that something really bad was going to happen that may aggravate my brain injury. Because I was now so desperate I was no longer saying please and thank you to the nurses but swearing at them in quite an aggressive manner. I was only doing this to get some help and at no time did I ever threaten to hit anyone. I thought that surely they would know about my history of mental illness and how lack of sleep affected it but it seemed not. As I was scared about injuring my head I was now walking along the corridor with a pillow across my forehead but the nurse seemed to be more concerned that this was blocking my vision than with the fact that I was having a full blown manic episode. I had asked the charge nurse if I could see a doctor but she had said that it could be some time before one was available. They did call my parents and I asked them to tell my Dad it was a Dundee United European game as I figured that Dad would know what I was referring to and drive through to Dundee as quickly as he could. I decided to wait in the quiet room until the doctor arrived. I was still shouting for the nurses to help me but only Dr Gentleman came in to see me and that was only to tell me that he did not accept any patients being aggressive to his staff. I could not understand his attitude as surely he realised that I was ill and I even mentioned Ann Gentleman who my Auntie thought might be a relative of his. I was basically pleading with him to help me and asking him what Ann would think about him just leaving me lying on the floor. Earlier that day on the news there had been a story about a nursing home down south called Winterbourne Gardens where several of the staff had been jailed for their mistreatment of patients under their care. Well I felt as if I was now in Winterbourne Gardens. I pulled the cushions of the sofa to enable me to lie on them as I was absolutely shattered and could not support my own body weight anymore. I was lying curled up on the cushions with nobody answering my cries for help when I noticed a white mug on the coffee table in front of me. I had decided by that point that the only way I was going to get help was if I managed to smash the window in the room and attract the attention of somebody outside. I picked up the mug and threw it as hard as I possibly could at the glass. There was a massive smashing noise and I thought that I had succeeded in breaking the window. Unfortunately it was only the mug that had smashed into a hundred tiny pieces. I had now decided in my head that even though I had just completed twenty years in hell with my Dystonia I was going to have to face another twenty years. I could not understand this as I had done nothing wrong but suddenly a clear thought entered my head. I was being punished for the sins of my father. This not only terrified me but made me very angry as enough was enough. Why should I pay for his sins when I had only tried to follow the path God had laid out for me.

Just then the door of the quiet room opened and standing there was a policeman who was surprised to see me in such distress. I felt as if I only had a short time to tell him about everything that was going on. I was no longer going to be punished for my father's sins so I told him my Dads registration, name and also that he would probably be driving through to Dundee at about one hundred and twenty miles an hour as we spoke. I also told him that I was having a manic episode and I had only thrown the mug at the window to attract attention from someone outside the hospital as the nursing staff had decided to leave me where I was for the past hour and it felt as if I was suddenly a patient in Winterbourne Gardens. The policeman's name was Simon Donaldson and his partner was called Kerry. Simon seemed to believe everything I was saying and he said that he would go and have a quick chat with the doctor. Now that five minutes he spent talking to the doctor was the longest five minutes of my life as I didn't know if he was going to come back again. Kerry popped her head in to reassure me that they were still there. She got me a cup of water as I was really thirsty and a tissue for my knee as a piece of the smashed mug had inadvertently cut it. I have no idea what was discussed between Simon and the doctor but eventually I was able to get to my feet and move out of the quiet room. I thanked Simon and Kerry for saving my life and said to Simon that he was definitely now going up to the spirit in the sky when he died! He said that he now wouldn't be able to get that tune out of his head for the rest of the day. They had another call to go to so they said goodbye but if required they would come back. I no longer felt abandoned so I told them that everything was now ok.

I made my way back to my bed because the trauma of the last hour had left me sapped of energy. I collapsed on to my bed and tried to rest. As I was resting Dr Mitch Stewart came to see me. As a psychiatrist he seemed to have a better understanding of my illness and what I was going through. He suggested that it may be in my best interests to get transferred to Murray Royal Hospital in Perth. Now I knew they could give me enough medication to get me some sleep so I didn't really have to think about this suggestion for very long. I had also been in Murray Royal in 1998 and 2008 so it was a place that held no fears for me. My Mum was also part of the carers group so she had visited the new Moredun B ward that had just opened there and she seemed convinced that I would like my new surroundings. I told Mr Stewart that I would agree to be transferred as a voluntary patient. Initially I refused the option of having a nurse come through in the ambulance with me but eventually I decided that it would be nice to have Alan accompany me. I packed all my clothes, cards and other bits and pieces. It was beginning to feel like every time I moved hospitals I had acquired more and more stuff and I filled my rucksack and another bag. It was not long before the ambulance arrived. I gave Jane a very emotional hug as she had been very special in my care at the hospital. Even my dad gave her a hug which was very surprising as he was and never had been very tactile. It was a beautiful day so most of the patients were sitting at the tables outside the front door. In my mind I thought that they could feel that I was placed on this Earth to help them but of course they couldn't but they were still very upset to see me go. Ann and June gave me a couple of big teary hugs although most of the tears were coming from me. I shook hands with Chris and Colin. When shaking hands with Chris I used my left hand and he used his left too as we both had problems with opposite sides so it was more natural to shake hands this way. I gave Evelyn a kiss on the cheek after I had given Jim a big hug and the only thing he said was "don't forget us". I felt he was asking for my help and as he and the other patients were my friends I had no intention of letting them down. The ambulance slowly pulled away from the entrance and I waved goodbye to another chapter in my life.

CHAPTER TEN

I made sure my seatbelt was on before we set off as I was not in the mood for taking any risks now as I was starting to feel as if I may be getting closer to the end of one journey but also nearer to the beginning of another. Alan, the bus driver and I had a good laugh on the way up to the hospital. The driver was kind enough to play a couple of CD's on the way up the road. I asked Alan to apologise to the other nurses in the brain clinic, when he got back, for my bad language but I really had no control over my outbursts at that stage. He accepted my apology. The journey from Dundee to Perth took about forty minutes but I was now so excited to see what the future would bring time was no longer important to me.

We arrived at the spanking new Moredun B ward building. The driver offered to help me off the bus with my second bag but I rather emotionally said that I was going to walk in under my own steam and walk out under my own steam too. I remember that I waited for three young ladies to walk out of the front door before I went in. They were very attractive and I thought to myself I'm going to like it here! We walked along several very long corridors but they were so bright compared with the old unit that I had been in five years ago. We finally got to the front door of the actual ward which was locked. I was met by a couple of nurses who knew me from my previous admissions but I could not remember their names. I entered the ward and was shown to a table in the canteen where I met Dr Jack or Mary as she introduced herself. She was very tall and extremely attractive.

I then had to go through the by now, all too common admission process. This went on for some time and by the end of it Alan and I didn't even have time for the coffee and cake we had promised each other when we left Dundee. I said thanks and goodbye to Alan and was shown to my room which was a complete contrast to the rather drab rooms we got on the old Moredun B ward. Everyone now got their own single room with en-suite facilities and my room also had a nice view over the garden and also the hills in the distance. I already felt a lot safer here than I had done in the brain clinic and I was more than happy to unpack my belongings. The get well soon cards gave the room a bit more of a homely feeling. The nurse came in and confiscated my sharps but I still haven't worked out how you actually get the blades out of a Gillette Mac 3 razor to enable you to cut your wrists. I was actually surprised that I was allowed to keep my belt and shoe laces as these were usually locked away too.

After I had checked in I started to meet a lot of nurses that recognised me from my last admission in 2008 but I found it difficult to remember all of their names. The senior charge nurse was still Phil which was very pleasing as I really liked her. Unfortunately a patient I remembered from five years ago was also on the ward. He was in a wheelchair and his wife was in another ward on the hospital grounds, but this didn't give him the right to be so rude to fellow patients and staff. He had been a nasty piece of work five years ago and nothing had changed yet you would have thought we were best of mates by the way he greeted me as a long lost pal.

I made my way through to the canteen for dinner. All the food was pretty good, now that I had got my taste buds back after giving up smoking. I did notice in the dining room that one of the patients had taken an instant dislike to me as he seemed to think that I much preferred the sound of my own voice as to anyone else's. This was a good wakeup call as even if you wanted to be friends with everybody you were not always going to be everyone's cup of tea. The canteen was spilt into men and women and the two men who were sitting at my table were very nice. We had a nice meal and a good laugh.

My recollection of the first few days back in Murray Royal is not that great because I was still trying to catch up on nine days of sleep deprivation and also readjust to life back on a psychiatric ward. The good thing was that I felt I was now in the correct place to get treatment for my manic episode and with increased medication I could feel myself getting stronger every day. I was still fearful of either falling off my bed at night or banging my head of the wall in my room so the nurses turned my bed around so that it was now parallel to the wall and they also gave me extra pillows that I could put on the ground in case I fell out of the bed.

Most of the nurses remembered me from my last visit and as I was usually well behaved I seemed to have made quite a good impression first time round. There were a couple of new younger nurses who were gorgeous. One was called Chloe and the other Rhianon. Even though she was far too young for me if I had met Chloe on the outside I would definitely have tried to invite her out on a date! I quickly got back into the routine of the ward and my increased medication meant that I could now get some sleep. The first time I went to get my medication I forgot the golden rule of any psychiatric ward. Do not push in front of anyone when medication is getting handed out. Even if I did not push in on purpose I was reminded verbally in no uncertain terms that I better not do this again!

I was still waking up very early because I still felt that I had been asleep for twenty years with my Dystonia, so when I did wake up I wanted to make the most of each and every day. This meant that I was sometimes ready to have a shower at 4.30am. Now I knew this was very early but when I went to get some towels I was told it was too early even though I was forty two years old and the shower was in my room so it wasn't as if I was going to disturb anyone. I felt that I was old enough to decide when I could take a shower and also when we arrived on the ward we weren't given a rule book that prohibited showers before a certain time. If there had been a rule book then I would have abided by the rules but this was really the staff making up the rules as they went along which I didn't like. The other thing that would have helped on arrival was a map of the ward. It was a circular design and because of my blind spot my mind did not register rooms on the left of the ward which meant I spent the first few days on the ward walking round in circles!

It was probably about the third night on the ward when I was wakened by Chloe who was in my room, her face really close to mine, shouting "FIRE, FIRE"! Probably due to the medication I was taking it took some time for the words to register and that this wasn't a drill. Since my operation and the machine being switched on I had been having a bit of trouble releasing things from my left hand and so it was on this occasion that I proceeded to drag my duvet all the way along the corridor with Chloe screaming at me to let it go. I did eventually let it go but it has never been seen since so maybe one of the firemen picked it up.

I was still very conscious that the brain surgery had left my skull very fragile and therefore from time to time, usually just before medication, I would walk along the corridor with a pillow over the front of my head just in case I fell. The nursing staff were aware of these moments of anxiety and usually gave me my medication a little early to settle me down. However on one occasion the nurse with the keys for the drugs cabinet could not be found anywhere on the ward and I was getting more and more anxious with every passing second. I couldn't believe that there was only one set of keys in the first place as surely the location of the key holder could never be guaranteed. Eventually the key holder was found and I got my medication just in time. You may wonder what I mean when I say just in time or just in time for what? Well when I started to feel anxious like this it was always because I thought I was going to have to do something else to prove God existed and I became terrified that I would be asked to sacrifice myself again just as I had done in the psychiatric unit in America. Now the last thing I wanted to do was die as I had only started living but I knew if asked to do so I would not be able to refuse.

With this in mind on one night I got a really strong feeling that God was going to require something more from me and I didn't know if this would involve banging my fragile head of the walls in the ward. To protect myself I took a pillow with me just in case and also a belt. The belt was to tie the pillow tightly round my head just in case I did bang it off the wall. Now when the nurses see any patient with a belt in a psychiatric ward they automatically assume the worst so even though I didn't really know why there was a sudden panic to get this belt from me. I was now in front of the treatment rooms where we received our medication and a queue had already formed. A couple of nurses were already rushing towards me but it was in fact one of the patients who prised the belt away from me. The other amazing thing was that all the patients waiting for their medication allowed me to go first. It was as if they could feel my pain and knew that at that particular time my need was greater than theirs. It was a very humbling experience but I accepted their generosity and went in to get my medication first. I apologised to the staff for giving them a scare with the belt but Scott told me not to worry as he had realised what I was trying to do with the belt and it was definitely not to kill myself.

Now a few days after my admission to the ward Mum and Dad were visiting but although I loved seeing Mum I always felt uncomfortable with Dad as I realised that he had absolutely no understanding of mental illness. He had also bought me a Casio digital watch to enable me to tell the time when I was in Ninewells Hospital. Due to my blind spot reading the time on a normal clock face was now difficult as the brain was having difficulty recording the left hand side of the clock face. Dad had put the watch on my wrist and initially it didn't feel at all tight. However after the episode in the quiet room at the brain clinic my skin had been visible through the small holes on the watch strap it was on so tight around my wrist. I felt that God was trying to tell me that Dad was evil and was not to be trusted. Even though I felt that I was getting closer and closer to my journeys end this made me more and more scared that something could go wrong. I had decided that it was a battle of Good against Evil and I actually told Dad this but when I did he just said "and I presume I'm the evil". Now this confirmed in my mind that Dad did represent Evil so I decided that if I was going to get better quickly then I couldn't see him on the ward anymore. I explained this to him face to face leaving out the part about good versus evil and just reinforcing the fact that I had to think of myself now even if that meant I might hurt his feelings. A few days later when my brother Scott was due to visit I said to Mum that we all, including Dad, could sit round the table and talk everything through without any confrontation but Dad decided not to come.

I was now getting better every day as I caught up on all that lost sleep. I even managed to sleep through the entire opening ceremony for the Olympics on a sofa in the pool room. I had my weekly meeting with Dr Curran, Dr Jack and Dr Ocean and they decided that as I was progressing so well that I could have a three hour pass each day. This pass could be taken as one lump sum of three hours or separate periods up to a maximum of three hours. This was great because it meant that I could go to the café at the front of the building for a bacon roll and a coffee for breakfast. More importantly it meant I could take a complete break from the ward for five minutes or three hours depending on how I felt at the time.

I was very relieved to finally get these passes as it had felt like I was being overlooked when it came to time away from the ward. Several other patients who in my opinion were much more fragile and vulnerable than me were already out on day and weekend passes and I did feel that the nurses had not even got to the root of their problems. This was mainly due to a lack of time but also because many mental health patients often see the doctors and nurses as the enemy and therefore find it difficult to open up to them. As far as I was concerned then I was one of them so they felt they could trust me with most of their problems.

This was certainly the case with Ian who was an alcoholic. He was due to be discharged in a couple of days which amazed me as there was no way he was ready to go back to his old life. Ian was one of the nicest men you could ever meet but if anything he was too nice. This meant he could be easily manipulated even if he didn't realise it. Ian smoked a lot yet he would be prepared to give his last cigarette to Jimmy even though Jimmy had cigarettes left but was just taking advantage of this patient's generous nature. The terrible thing was that on the outside Ian's brother was also an alcoholic but his brother would take every last penny of his giro cheque every two weeks and Ian wouldn't see a penny. This would mean that until Ian had learned how to say no there was very little chance of him being able to stay of the drink on the outside and also lead a normal life. He spoke about the fact that he was still a virgin despite being in his forties and never having had a girlfriend. I sincerely hope that Ian has managed to prise himself away from the nasty claws of his brother and the evil drink but I don't hold out much hope. It is even sadder that after all these years Ian had finally plucked up the courage to ask for our help and yet because we didn't have the time to listen we would be sending him back into the arms of evil.

Probably the patient that affected me most was Alice. Now her name wasn't Alice but this is what I had been calling her on the ward so I will leave it as this because Alice was the name of Bill's wife and Bill had been a very good friend to me in and out of Murray Royal until he finally succeeded in taking his own life several years ago. I had also felt that Bill was watching over me while I was on the ward to make sure nothing bad happened. Now one evening I asked Alice how she was feeling and I could tell by the shake of her head that it wasn't good. We went into the ladies TV room for a chat as there was nobody in there. I shut the door behind me and pulled up a chair directly in front of Alice's. Alice's husband of forty years had died five days before her admission and in those five days she had attempted to take her own life four times. Amazingly Alice was going to be discharged tomorrow on a weekend pass back to the house where she and her husband had shared so many happy memories. I thought going back to her own house might not be doing her recovery any good so I offered her my spare room when I got out. I have subsequently learned from another friend that if someone doesn't face their old home after bereavement then there is every possibility that they will never go back. I suppose it's almost like getting back on the horse but in this case having the courage to open that front door again. Alice told me that she could not carry on without her beloved husband as she was broken inside. I could feel her pain but as I explained, as the tears fell down both our cheeks, I could not take this pain away. There was no point giving her false hope either so I told her that the pain wouldn't get any better tomorrow or for a very long time and it would probably never completely go. A nurse walked past the door and Alice suddenly became very anxious as she didn't want anyone to know that she was feeling this way. In fact she made me promise that I would not tell any of the nurses or doctors. I promised. Alice was upset that the tears were rolling down my cheeks too but I think those tears were helping me release some of my own emotions that had been bottled up for too long. Even though I was terrified that Alice would indeed take her own life on discharge I also knew that I couldn't betray her trust as I knew that I could not save all of the people all of the time. We ended the conversation with a big hug.

I did try to come and see Alice on the ward after my own discharge but as I didn't have her last name I wasn't allowed to speak to her in person. I left a message with a nurse so that she could phone me if she wanted a visit but obviously I don't know if this message was passed on but she never called. I was out the other day with Bill's wife, the real Alice, and over coffee she told me about a lady that had thrown herself of Kinnoull Hill. My heart sank thinking it might be the lady from the ward but as Alice continued I realised that it was another poor soul who had come to the conclusion that the future or the past was too dark to go on in the present.

The doctor who was looking after me when I was on the ward was Dr Curran although Dr Jack and Dr Ocean also sat in during the weekly meetings about my care. It was decided that my progress was such that I could be discharged on Monday. Before this could happen my flat had to be assessed by occupational therapy to make sure that I would be able to cope with the weakness in my left side when I went home. Rhona and I went to the flat and it was agreed that I needed a seat over the bath for taking a shower and a bar next to the toilet as well as an additional rail on the right of my inside stairs. These would take a couple of weeks so they wouldn't be in by the time I got home on Monday. This wasn't a big deal as getting home was the most important thing as I could always wash myself at the sink.

I had been doing my own clothes washing in the ward for the past few weeks but you always had to get a nurse to open the laundry room door as it was usually locked. On one such occasion I had got the nurse to open the door so I could transfer my clothes into the tumble drier. Now my Nike golf T shirts only need twenty minutes in the drier but this nurse thought that you had to put the machine on for at least forty five minutes. I don't think she was very happy that I knew a bit more about the drying machines than she did. This was shown to be the case later on that evening at dinner as I went up to ask her for two napkins and she laughed and said 'two nappies'! Now I did not find this very funny so I went and told Phil what had happened. Phil agreed with me and said she would have a word with the nurse in question which she did. The nurse then came rushing out of the food service area to say that she had misheard me and that the other nurse at the counter had also thought I said nappies. She then suddenly changed her story to say it was just a bit of banter but I pointed out that I didn't think it was very funny. The nurse then apologised and I accepted her apology. I had never liked this nurse but in life you were never going to like all of the people all of the time.

I now couldn't wait to get home as I think I had spent just about as much time in hospital as I could take for one year. Mum came to pick me up on the Monday and I was ready and waiting. I went to get my bag from my room but too my horror when I returned Mum was speaking to the nurse who had made the comment about the nappies. Now when you have spent a few weeks on a psychiatric ward and then it is finally your discharge date the last thing you want is to be held up especially by your Mum talking to one of the nurses you don't trust or like. Mum seemed to want to clarify my discharge details but off course she could have done this by asking me what they were instead of asking this nurse. I basically let Mum know that

I was leaving now and nothing was going to hold me up. She finally got the message and as I said three weeks earlier when I walked into the ward I picked up my rucksack and walked out of the ward. I knew that this was only another small chapter of my life closing and that a new more joyous, more exciting and more rewarding journey was just on the other side of the automatic doors but at least I was a free man again. I now knew that I could go forward and try and use the gift that God had given me. To prove that God exists.

I had no idea how I was going to do this but I felt sure that God would guide me just as he had guided me to this point in my life and therefore despite having no doubt about the size and importance of the task I did feel that it was achievable. As I write this the doorbell has just rung and two Jehovah witnesses Claire and Penny have just handed me this month's magazine which is centred on the subject 'What is God's name'. Obviously they believe that his name is Jehovah but even though this is mentioned in the bible I don't think it would matter if we called God Jim, Paul, Scott, Mark or anything else for that matter just as long as we realise that he is God creator of all, saviour of all who sacrificed his own Son for all our sins. Let's just call him God to prevent confusion but if you have your own pet name for him then that's ok too.

The most important thing is that you recognise him every day and in everything you do in your life. He is everywhere and in everything we do. He lives through us so make sure you make his life a joyous one as remember the pain suffered on the cross for you. It is incumbent on all of us to live our lives for Jesus as he lives his life through us now and we have to make sure we live like he would every day. Even Jesus wasn't perfect so don't think that this is impossible. Only he could perform miracles but there is no reason that your own miracle can't be living your life as the best person you can be each and every day. Now this doesn't mean you can't have any fun as

Jesus is all about fun and the joy of life. In fact your life will be filled with more fun if you let God in. I guarantee it as he has guaranteed it. The card I picked up at the church last Sunday said it all:-

Be joyful always
Pray continually
Give thanks in all circumstances,
 As this is God's will,
For you in Christ Jesus

If you live your life as it says on the card then you will feel the joy of the Lord on a daily basis. Now God knows that we are not perfect and we will fall of the horse or even the wagon every now and again but as long as we dust ourselves of and try again tomorrow then he will always love you. It is never too late to change either so do not despair if your life so far has been some distance from the straight and narrow. We all make mistakes and if you have read this book you will know that I have made some whoppers but I know God still loves me and for that I'm thankful. I just pray that you too can find your way to him or maybe he like me has found you when you needed him most because miracles do happen and they can happen to anybody. I have no idea why he came to my rescue that night in 1998 but he did and I know he wants me to tell you nothing is impossible if you believe in God.

God Bless

THE END